SIMPLY *Delicious* RECIPES FOR DIABETICS

CHRISTINE ROBERTS
JENNIFER MCDONALD
MARGARET COX

Avery Publishing Group
Garden City Park, New York

The information presented in this book should not be construed as a substitute for professional medical advice. In any situation in which you have questions regarding the appropriateness of this information, always consult your health care provider.

Cover Design: William Gonzalez and Rudy Shur
Text Illustrations: John Wincek
Typesetter: Bonnie Freid

Cataloging-in-Publication Data

Roberts, Christine L., 1945-
  Simply delicious recipes for diabetics: simple and flavorful
dishes from appetizers to desserts / by Christine Roberts, Jennifer
McDonald, and Margaret Cox.
  p. cm.
  Includes index.
  ISBN 0-89529-688-8

  1. Diabetes—Diet therapy—Recipes. I. McDonald, Jennifer.
II. Cox, Margaret R., 1944- III. Title.

RC662.R63 1996   641.5'6314
                                    QBI96-20336

10 9 8 7 6 5 4 3

Contents

Acknowledgments

There are a number of people who have helped and encouraged us in the writing of this book.

We'd especially like to thank Jacqui Roberts for undertaking the difficult task of analyzing the recipes and meal plans.

The expertise, advice, and hard work of René Gordon, our Australian publisher, and her assistants Joy Bowers, Joslin Guest, and Des Carroll have made this book a reality. The splendid color photography is the work of Ann Creber, Lyn Zeeng, and Lynda Patullo and we appreciate their skill and creativity.

We'd also like to thank Cynthia Miles, R.D., and Sandra Woodruff, R.D., diabetes nutrition consultants, their help in reviewing this manuscript for the U.S. audience.

Most importantly, we thank our families, and especially our husbands Noel Roberts, Michael Hall, and Jack Cox—without their support, patience, encouragement, and understanding, we could never have completed *Simply Delicious Recipes for Diabetics*.

Christine Roberts

Jennifer McDonald

Margaret Cox

Introduction

As dietitians working with people with diabetes, we are constantly being asked to provide individuals with all the information they need about diet, cooking and eating. In the course of our work over the years, we were very aware how little simple, straightforward and up-to-date information there was about the relationship between food and diabetes.

Many people with diabetes don't have enough detailed, yet easily understood, information about the way in which the food they eat affects the control of diabetes, and this makes them unsure of how to plan or prepare their meals.

In the past few years, there have been major changes in the principles of eating for people with diabetes. Where in the past, people with diabetes were treated as being different, today we realize that the ideal diet for everyone is perfect for people with diabetes too.

Clearly there was a need for a book that explained simply the relationship between diabetes and food, laid out the guidelines needed for good management today, and included delicious and healthy recipes ideal for everyone, not just those with diabetes.

Simply Delicious does just that. Through this book we hope that you will have more confidence in your ability to maintain good health and enjoy the pleasures of the table.

Knowledge Is Sweet

More and more people are being diagnosed with diabetes. It is estimated that the number of people with diabetes mellitis in the United States is approximately 6.5 million, 90% with NIDDM (non-insulin dependent diabetes mellitis), and 10% with IDDM (insulin dependent diabetes mellitis).

Diabetes mellitus is not new. It may be as old as humanity. Certainly, it has been with us throughout recorded history, but only in 1921 did we learn to treat it with some effectiveness. And only in the past decade have we devised a new way of eating for people with diabetes. In the past 70 or so years, diabetes has changed from being a life-threatening condition to one that requires a change of lifestyle and, where necessary, medication.

WHERE TO GO FOR FURTHER HELP

If you or one of your family members are one of the 6.5 million who have been told they have diabetes mellitis, you will find that there are many resources that you can use in order to learn more about your condition, to put you in touch with support groups, and to help make your lifestyle adjustments easier. The following information should be helpful in helping you to locate those resources closest to you.

Dietitians

- Your state branch of the American Dietetic Association.
- Look under "Dietitian" or "Nutritionist" in the Yellow Pages or other telephone directory.
- Ask your local doctor if he or she knows of a particular dietitian to refer you to.
- Contact your community health center.
- Telephone your local hospital.
- Inquire at your state or community health department.

American Diabetes Association (ADA)

American Diabetes Association is the national coordinating organization providing a unique partnership between consumers—the people with diabetes—research organizations, doctors and other health professionals with a special interest in diabetes.

Look under American Diabetes Association in your telephone directory. American Diabetes Association will provide information on the following:

- Member organizations and the services they provide
- Diabetes education programs
- Diabetes camps
- National magazine *Diabetes Forecast*
- Additional membership advantages

What Is Diabetes?

You need to know what diabetes is before you can take an active part in managing your own health care.

"Diabetes" comes from the ancient Greek word for "siphon," referring to the large amount of sugar-containing urine passed by people with uncontrolled diabetes, and "mellitus" for the characteristic sweet taste of the urine. **Diabetes (more accurately diabetes mellitus) is simply too much sugar in the blood.**

This sugar is in the form of **glucose**. Diabetes occurs when the system which controls the amount of glucose in the blood no longer works properly.

But where does it all begin? **Everyone** has glucose in their blood all the time. It provides energy (or fuel) to keep the body working, much like the gas in a car.

WHERE DOES GLUCOSE COME FROM?

Glucose comes from the food we eat. When we eat carbohydrate (sugars and starches), our bodies convert it into glucose.

Some of the Foods Rich in Carbohydrate:

- Breads, cereals, and crackers
- Legumes/beans (such as dried peas, beans, and lentils)
- Starchy vegetables (such as potatoes)
- Rice and pasta
- Fruit
- Milk
- Sugar
- Foods with sugar added, such as cakes, cookies, candy, sweetened soft drinks and canned fruit.

The digestive system breaks down carbohydrate to make glucose. The glucose is then absorbed into the bloodstream directly from the digestive tract or gut.

What Happens to the Glucose?

The blood carries the glucose to your body tissues (for instance, your brain, lungs, heart, liver, kidneys, and muscles). There, the glucose passes from your blood into the tiny cells that make up body tissues, but the only way in which this can happen is with the help of the hormone *insulin*. On the wall of each tiny cell are special key holes or receptor sites. The insulin attaches itself to the glucose in the blood and locks itself into the receptor site in much the same way as you would use a key to open a door. This allows the glucose to pass through the cell wall into the cell where it is used for fuel.

Insulin is produced by the pancreas, a small gland that lies behind the stomach. Scattered throughout the pancreas are clusters of specialized cells, the Islets of Langerhans, which make and store insulin, and then release it into the bloodstream as needed. The pancreas, despite its small size, also produces digestive juices which help your body break down food as it passes through the intestines.

After you have eaten, digested, and absorbed food containing carbohydrate, the amount of glucose in your blood increases. In response to this, the pancreas releases the correct amount of insulin into your blood to carry the extra glucose into the cells. The amount of glucose in your blood then returns to its pre-meal level. At least, that's the way the system is supposed to work.

If you don't have diabetes, your blood glucose level never goes too high or too low, no matter how much or how little carbohydrate you eat. The system balances itself.

What Happens When Diabetes Develops?

When the body produces little or no insulin, or the insulin it does produce is unable to carry glucose into your body cells, you develop diabetes.

With your normal glucose regulating system out of order, your level of blood glucose keeps increasing. When it reaches a certain level, the body attempts to tackle the problem by passing the extra glucose out of your body via your urine. This is called 'glycosuria'—literally "glucose urine." Not surprisingly, with it can come symptoms such as:

- Passing large amounts of urine by day and night. This is called polyuria meaning "much urine," and nocturia meaning "night urine" as a way of getting rid of the excess sugar.
- Feeling very thirsty most of the time and having a dry mouth, the result of the large urine output.
- Drinking excessively (polydipsia) in response to thirst.
- Excessive tiredness due to the lack of available fuel to the cells.

- Losing weight because the normal fuel, glucose, is not available and the body breaks down fat stores.

- Itchiness and infections resulting from bacteria feeding on the extra glucose in blood and urine.

- Blurring of vision due to the effect of the high blood glucose on the fluid levels in the eye.

A medical examination will then reveal a high blood glucose level, in other words, a diagnosis of diabetes.

> *A high blood glucose level is known as hyperglycemia, from "hyper," meaning excessive and "glycemia" for sugar in the blood.*

What is a Normal Blood Glucose Level?

A normal blood glucose range for a person without diabetes is between 80 and 100 mg/dL.

A fasting blood glucose level greater than 140 mg/dL or a random (that is, not fasting), glucose level greater than 200 mg/dL confirms a diagnosis of diabetes. (World Health Organization recommendations.)

Note that fasting blood glucose is checked when you have been without food or drink for 10-12 hours. A random test can be taken at any time, regardless of whether you have eaten or not.

TYPES OF DIABETES

There are two main types of diabetes:

- Insulin-Dependent Diabetes Mellitus (IDDM)—Type 1
- Non-Insulin Dependent Diabetes Mellitus (NIDDM)—Type 2

Insulin–Dependent Diabetes Mellitus (IDDM)—Type 1

IDDM can develop at any age, but usually does so in childhood, during the teens or in early adulthood. What causes it is still unknown, but it may be caused by a virus which leads to the destruction of the Islets of Langerhans within the pancreas. Whatever the cause, the pancreas stops making insulin and symptoms usually appear quickly and severely.

If not treated promptly, your blood glucose level rises. As the glucose cannot get into the cells, your body begins burning up its fat stores too quickly (ketosis) and your breath smells of acetone. You may vomit, become dehydrated and feel drowsy. Left untreated, you will eventually lapse into a coma.

About 10 percent of all people with diabetes have this type. The treatment is a combination of insulin injections and a healthy diet, like the one we present in this book. It is necessary to inject insulin, because if it were taken by mouth it would be destroyed by digestive juices long before it could be absorbed and used.

Non-Insulin Dependent Diabetes Mellitus (NIDDM)—Type 2

This is by far the more common of the two types of diabetes. It develops slowly and symptoms, if any, are likely to be less extreme than with IDDM. The only sign may be a high blood glucose level (hyperglycemia) picked up on routine testing by your doctor.

NIDDM usually develops in people over the age of 40. It accounts for about 90 percent of all cases. There is often a family history of diabetes.

A number of factors may influence the development of NIDDM, most importantly:

Family history, age, weight, stress, alcohol abuse, and inactivity.

With this type of diabetes, the pancreas makes some insulin, but not enough. Alternatively, excess body fat stops the insulin from carrying glucose into the body's cells.

Treatment for NIDDM is simply a healthy diet and exercise. If this is not enough to control the blood glucose, then oral medication or insulin may be given. For the overweight person with this type of diabetes, **losing weight is the most important part of treatment**.

Even with well-controlled diabetes, insulin or extra oral medication may be needed during periods of illness, after surgery or emotional distress.

Diabetes Medication/Pills and How They Work:
Diabetes medications (oral hypoglycemic agents) help lower your blood glucose level. They don't contain insulin, but they do help the body make more insulin or help you use the insulin you have more effectively.

What happens if diabetes remains uncontrolled?

If your blood glucose level remains high or fluctuates excessively over a period, this may damage the blood vessels that supply your eyes, kidneys, heart and other organs and nerves, especially in your legs and feet. Learning how to manage your diabetes and to achieve good control is the best way to avoid these complications.

Managing Diabetes Today

Essentially, good management of diabetes focuses on three major approaches:

- Diet
- Diet and diabetes medication
- Diet and insulin injections

Exactly which approach is most beneficial for you will depend on what type of diabetes you have, your weight, age and your blood glucose level. Regular exercise makes an important difference to all people with diabetes and to your sense of well-being and general health.

There are two other important guidelines which will keep you fit and in good health:

- **Regular monitoring of your blood or urine glucose levels** helps you get to know your body and how it is coping with diabetes. It shows you the effect food, exercise and medication have on your blood glucose level (BGL), and helps you adjust them as necessary.
- **Regular visits to your doctor, dietitian and/or diabetes educator**—your partners in ongoing health care.

WHAT CAN DIET DO FOR DIABETES?

Food is important in keeping healthy, whether we have diabetes or not. However, most people don't pay enough attention to their basic nutritional needs. Diabetes highlights the importance of a well-balanced eating pattern.

If you have diabetes, there are three important benefits to be had from a nutritionally sound diet:

- First, it helps you achieve and maintain good control of your blood glucose level.
- Second, it helps you regulate your body weight.
- Third, it helps prevent or delay the onset of any of the long-term problems linked with diabetes.

THE GOLDEN RULES FOR DIABETES

The way to keep healthy now and in the future is to follow these Golden Rules:

- **Understand your diabetes and how to manage it.** Ask questions. Don't be shy or worry that you seem "stupid" or are being a bother. No matter how "silly" your question, ask it. And keep on asking until you are entirely satisfied that you understand your diabetes and know what to do to manage it. If, like so many people, you tend to go blank when seeing the dietitian, doctor or diabetes educator, sit down before your visit and write out all your questions and concerns. Take your list with you and go through it item by item.

  These people are often busy and, if you need extra time, make an appointment for a less busy time. Alternatively, ask for a double appointment. Make sure you understand exactly what the prescribed treatment is supposed to do, and exactly how to follow it. You can also take a parent, friend or partner to help you remember what was said.

- **Keep your blood glucose level under control.** The best way of doing this is to eat sensibly, exercise regularly and take your medication correctly. Check your blood glucose levels regularly and have your doctor or diabetes educator do this at regular intervals.

- **If you are overweight, make losing weight a goal.** If you are slim, stay slim. There is no magic to losing weight. Basically, you need to make sure that you eat fewer calories than your body burns up. You probably know whether you are eating too much, but if you are unsure of how to cut down on calories without losing out on good nutrition, look at the meal plans in this book.

  Once you are slim, keep a careful watch on what you eat; it's all a matter of balance. You need to eat just enough to fuel your body through its normal daily routine, so concentrate on those things that provide your body with enough nutrients to keep it functioning perfectly. Remember, you can do this and still enjoy varied and tasty meals.

- **Be as physically active as possible**, keeping in mind your age, general health and your ability to exercise. This is not a call to becoming a super-athlete; you can keep fit simply by taking a brisk walk around the block twice a day. You may prefer to swim a few laps, play tennis, ride your bicycle or walk to the local shops instead of driving. But whatever exercise you choose, and whatever level of physical activity you find most comfortable, make it a regular part of your life. The benefits are immense.

Understanding the Principles of Good Nutrition

Food is an important part of life—it is a necessity and it should be a pleasure. Diabetes need not change either of these aspects.

What we eat is a very individual matter. It's one of those areas where personal choice is allowed a wide expression. How you feel at any particular moment, your tastes, your cultural background and lifestyle all have an effect on your food choices.

The enjoyment we get from food should be matched by its value as a source of nourishment. It's the sort of thing we all are becoming more aware of, but may well ignore. However, when you develop diabetes, you have the opportunity to reappraise what you eat and improve your eating habits with immediate and significant benefits.

Foods provide a range of different textures, flavors, colors, and nutritional values, and eating a variety will ensure the best combination for good health. The nutrients in food include protein, fat, carbohydrate, vitamins, minerals, fiber, and water, all of which are essential for continued good health. It may be of help to know what these different nutrients do, and why they are vital.

Protein

- Is an important part of all body tissues, enzymes, hormones and the immune system.
- You need protein for body growth and repair.
- Has only a small role as a body fuel.
- The richest sources are meat, poultry, fish, seafood, dairy products, eggs, nuts, seeds, and beans. You don't have to eat huge quantities of protein to meet your body needs.

Fat

- Provides fuel to keep the body working.

- Plays an important part in insulating and protecting the body's organs and other tissues.
- Transports other nutrients into and around the body.
- You need very small amounts daily to perform these important tasks. Major sources include butter, margarine, oils, meat, milk, cream and cheese.

Carbohydrate

- Is the most important fuel source for all body tissues, especially the brain.
- Plays an important part in many body functions.
- Comes in two main forms—sugars and starches. Sugars are found naturally in fruit, milk and honey, and are added as sweeteners to many foods such as candy, cakes, soft drinks, and jams. You find starches in breads, cereals, grains, vegetables, and beans/legumes.

Vitamins

- Help the body produce fuel from carbohydrate, fat and protein.
- Work in combination with protein in growth and repair of body tissues.
- Play an essential part in body functions.

There are two types:

- Water-soluble vitamins, that is, vitamin C and all B vitamins, which are found widely in foods including fruits, vegetables, cereals, milk, and meat.
- Fat-soluble vitamins—A, D, E and K—which are found in animal fats such as butter, other dairy products, meat, vegetable oils and margarines, wholegrain products, nuts and seeds.

Minerals

- Form a major part of bones, teeth and body fluids such as blood.
- Play an essential part in body functions such as heart beat, muscle contraction, and in nervous system and fluid balance.
- Occur widely in foods such as meat and fish, milk and cheese, fruits, vegetables and cereal products.

Fiber

- Used to be called "roughage" and is the part of plant foods which is not broken down by the digestive juices.

- Has several tasks, including keeping the digestive tract in good shape. In other words, it keeps our bowels functioning regularly and easily.

- Also helps fill the stomach, satisfies our appetite and helps to limit over-eating.

- Delays the onset of hunger by slowing both digestion and the rate at which our body absorbs nutrients. In particular, from the point of view of a person with diabetes, it slows the rate of absorption of carbohydrate from the gut, thereby helping to control the blood glucose level.

- Is invaluable in your diet. Eat lots of it. Good sources of fiber include wholegrain breads and cereals, fruits, vegetables and beans/legumes.

Water

- Is an essential part of every body function. About two-thirds of the body is water.

- We lose between one and three litres of water every day through the lungs and in urine, feces and sweat. The body can survive only for a few days without replacing this loss.

- Is the best drink for health. Don't wait until you're thirsty. Drink at least six to eight cups of water a day, and you will feel the benefit.

Food as a Fuel Source

Food is the energy source or fuel that keeps our bodies working. The energy supplied by any food is measured in calories. Energy comes from three particular nutrients in our food. We have ranked them in order of importance: carbohydrate; then fat; lastly protein.

Alcohol provides concentrated energy, but it isn't usually considered a nutrient and certainly isn't essential.

GUIDELINES TO CHOOSING FOOD

A good guide for choosing a healthy diet is set out in the following dietary guidelines. Follow these guidelines and you will be on the way to managing your health and your diabetes. The first five are particularly important if you have diabetes:

- Eat plenty of bread and cereals (preferably wholegrain), beans/legumes, vegetables and fruit.

- Limit your sugar intake.
- Limit your fat intake.
- Limit the amount of alcohol you drink.
- Control your weight.

But don't ignore the rest. Here they are:

- Choose a nutritious diet from a variety of foods.
- Cut back on salt.
- Encourage breastfeeding.
- Drink plenty of water.

And for women, teenage girls, athletes and vegetarians be sure to have enough iron and calcium to meet your additional needs.

In this section, we will explain why these guidelines are important to you.

EAT PLENTY OF WHOLEGRAIN BREADS AND CEREALS, BEANS, FRUITS, AND VEGETABLES

These foods offer a number of benefits, and should make up the bulk of your diet. They contain plenty of carbohydrate and fiber, vitamins and minerals and, if you eat them regularly, they will actually help control your diabetes. They will also help you control your weight because they are satisfying and bulky.

Important: Be sure to include the appropriate amount (as planned by your dietitian or physician) of high-carbohydrate, high-fiber food (as shown next) in every meal. If you are young and/or active, your carbohyrate requirements will be much higher than a sedentary adult's. You may find that you need more carbohydrate at meals and/or high carbohydrate snacks to ensure you have enough carbohydrate in your body all through the day.

Rather than using accurately weighed or measured foods we have used average servings as a basis for carbohydrate intake. Experience has shown that as long you are **consistent** this can give you good control and make life easier.

We have used 1 slice of bread as a standard but you can increase your servings according to your individual needs.

Cereals

Include bread, crackers, breakfast cereals, rice, wheat, barley, oats, buckwheat, rye, pasta (such as spaghetti and noodles).

1 serving	= 1 slice of bread	= 4–6 dry crackers
	= ¾ cup of cereal	= ½ cup of cooked pasta
	= ½ cup of cooked rice	

Beans/Legumes

Include dried beans (such as red kidney beans, black-eyed, lima, haricot, cannellini, and soy beans), peas (such as split peas and chick peas), and lentils.

1 serving   = ½ cup, cooked

Vegetables

Starchy vegetables include potatoes, sweet potatoes, corn, yams, and winter squash.

1 serving   = ½ cup, cooked
              = 1 medium potato

Vegetables, other than the starchy ones listed above, are low in carbohydrate, but high in fiber, and are a particularly rich source of minerals and vitamins. You should include plenty of them in your daily diet together with starchy vegetables.

Fruit

Include all varieties.

1 serving   = 1 medium piece of fresh fruit
              = ¾–1 cup stewed fruit

All About Carbohydrate and Fiber-Rich Food

Knowing about carbohydrate is important for you if you have diabetes. After all, carbohydrate breaks down into glucose, and balancing your blood glucose level is a vital part of your management.

It is useful for you to understand the difference between refined (simple) sugars such as sugar itself, and complex (unrefined) carbohydrate, such as in cereals, breads and beans/legumes.

Refined sugars such as table sugar are low in nutrients while providing energy, whereas complex carbohydrate-rich foods provide many essential nutrients and fiber as well as energy. Although fruit contains simple sugars, it also provides fiber and essential nutrients. Cereals, bread, legumes, starchy vegetables, and fruit should therefore form the basis of your eating plan.

Servings of different carbohydrate foods have different effects on the blood glucose levels, even when they provide the same amount of carbohydrate, with some causing a quicker and higher rise in blood glucose levels than others.

Foods are rated according to the effect they have on blood glucose levels. This is known as the **glycemic index.** Foods which cause a small rise in blood glucose levels have a low glycemic index number. Foods which cause a greater rise have a higher glycemic index number.

The best foods are those which have a low glycemic index number, provided they are also low in fat.

Many factors effect the glycemic index such as cooking, the amount of fat, the type of starch and fiber and the amount of processing.

What effect do these factors have?

Cooking - the more a food is cooked the easier it is for the body to break down the food and to absorb the carbohydrate and therefore the quicker the rise in blood glucose level.

Fat - foods high in fats often have a low glycemic index. This is due to the fat slowing down digestion. **However, high fat intake is not recommended for people with diabetes.**

Starches - different starches are broken down and absorbed at different rates.

Fiber - helps slow down the digestion and absorption of starches.

Processing - the more a food is processed the easier it is for the body to break down the food and absorb the carbohydrate.

The foods that offer the most benefits to people with diabetes in terms of glycemic index include:

- beans, all varieties

- oat, barley, and bran cereals

- breads containing large amounts of whole-grains such as pumpernickel, whole-grain rye, and wheat

- barley, buckwheat, bulgur

- basmati rice

- all pasta including spaghetti and noodles

- some fresh fruits such as apples, grapefruit, oranges, peaches, and plums

- some vegetables such as sweet potato and yam.

It is recommended that at least one serving of food of low glycemic index (as listed above) be included at each meal or one meal containing several foods of low glycemic index be included daily. This helps to even out swings in blood glucose levels and leads to better control.

This information is current, but research continues and there may be further changes.

Fiber

As mentioned earlier, fiber is important in helping control your blood glucose level and regulating bowel function. To maximize your fiber intake:

- Choose wholegrain breakfast cereals. For the best choices see the list on page 32.

- Replace white rice and pastas with brown rice and whole-grain pastas. You'll be delighted with how tasty they are.

- Use more beans in your cooking. Add them to soups, casseroles, salads, appetizers, and dips.

- Make sure you eat vegetables every day (including the starchy ones). Use them in salads, soups, meat dishes, and so on.

- Include at least two to three pieces of fruit in your daily eating plan. Preferably eat them fresh rather than cooked, and don't drink more than one **small** glass of fruit juice per day, as this is low in fiber.

- Leave vegetables and fruit unpeeled where possible, for maximum fiber.

LIMIT YOUR SUGAR INTAKE

An enormous number of the processed foods we eat contain added sugars. You will find sugar in many forms, some obvious, some less so, in many of the foods you buy such as cereals, crackers, cookies, canned fruit, soft drinks, candy, and chocolates. Sugars are high in calories but often are low in other nutrients. This means that they can add to your weight without providing any useful nourishment.

Diabetes does not mean a total ban on sugars. You can eat small amounts as part of meals without making your blood glucose level rise excessively. In practice, this means that a small amount of jam on whole wheat toast or a little sugar used in your whole wheat cake recipe will do no harm.

You can also train your palate to prefer far less sugar than we have become accustomed to in our western diet.

Hints to Help You Cut Down on Sugars

- Always check product labels. Read the section *Making Sense of Food Labels* (page 28).

- Avoid sugar in tea, coffee, or other beverages.

- Buy solid pack unsweetened canned fruit, fruit packed in water or natural juices, or artificially sweetened canned fruit instead of fruit canned in syrups.

- Water is the best thirst quencher. But if you must, use low-calorie soft drinks, and flavored mineral waters instead of the regular varieties.

- If you want gelatin desserts, use the low-calorie products.

- If you like jam, marmalade, or honey on your toast or bread, have some, but limit it to a small amount and forget the butter or margarine.

- In your cooking, look for recipes with very little or no sugar, fructose, or honey. Our recipes will give you a guide to just how little sugar or sweetness you need to make food delicious. Remember, too, that fruit is a good source of sweetness. In many of our recipes you will see that we use fruit and fruit juices in recipes that traditionally are made with sugar.

- Low-fat fruit yogurts are often surprisingly high in sugar. Choose those that are artificially sweetened or make your own by combining low-fat natural yogurt and your choice of fresh or stewed fruits.

- There are many excellent artificial sweeteners on the market. These may be used to replace sugar.

LIMIT YOUR FAT INTAKE

Fat is a taste-enhancer, and we have become used to eating far too much of it. Not only do we use it knowingly by frying foods or by ladling on the cream; we also eat a great deal of fat unknowingly in processed foods. It is sobering to realize that a 3 ounce package of potato chips contains 40% fat and 570 calories.

Because fat is the most concentrated form of energy we eat, there is a danger that a diet high in fats will add unnecessary calories. It may lead to weight gain.

Heart and circulation problems are often associated with a diet high in fats. Reduce your fat intake, and this may reduce your chances of developing such problems.

Remember that eating too much fat may have a direct effect on insulin activity in your body, causing an increase in your blood glucose level.

Just as you don't have to give up sweetness in your foods, you don't have to give up fats altogether. **It is important, however, that you limit your intake.** Cutting back begins in the kitchen, and continues at the table.

Hints to Help You Use Less Fat

- Select lean cuts of meat and remove skin and fatty deposits from poultry.

- Use the absolute minimum oil or fat in cooking. If possible, don't use any added fat at all.

- When you must use fat, use a brush to spread a thin layer of fat onto your pan, or use a cooking spray.

- Grill or roast meat on a rack to allow the fat to drip away.

- For soups and casseroles, drop meat into boiling water to seal it rather than browning it in fat or oil.

- Spread butter or margarine very thinly on bread and crackers, or leave it off. Use low-fat ricotta, low-fat cottage cheese, or a small amount of low-fat cream cheese as a spread instead.

- Use low-fat dairy products in preference to the regular varieties.

- Use "no-oil," "low-oil," or "low-calorie" salad dressings instead of oily ones or mayonnaise. Better still, use lemon juice or vinegar with herbs to add zest to your salads. Turn to our *Dressings* section (page 186) for ideas.

- Learn to use fresh or dried herbs and spices to add flavor to food instead of butter or oil.

- Avoid adding oil or fat to vegetables during or after preparation. For instance, when you mash potatoes or other vegetables, don't add butter, margarine or cream. Use low-fat milk. Wrap your vegetables in foil with herbs, or try dry baking them in the oven in their own skins.
- If you like sour cream as a vegetable dressing, use low-fat cottage cheese or low-fat natural yogurt instead.
- Use our recipe for Creamy Whipped Topping (see page 192) instead of cream on desserts.

Our recipes reflect our recommendations; we use fat, where necessary, but sparingly. The recipes will convince you that you can eat wonderful, nutritious food and still cut down on fat.

Protein

Protein foods often contain fat, so be aware of this when you make choices. Consider the following:

MEAT, POULTRY, FISH

Protein is important to a healthy eating plan and you should include some every day. Many people eat far too much. You only need one or two small servings of protein daily.

By a small serving, we mean about 3 oz of cooked meat or fish. To give you some idea of what this means, 3 oz of steak is a piece about the size of an average hamburger patty. If in doubt, at first weigh your meats or fish, or ask your butcher or fish store to weigh them for you.

When choosing protein foods, select those which are lower in fat, such as:

- **Lean** beef, veal, pork or lamb
- Chicken or turkey **without skin**
- Fish and seafood

To be classified as lean, meat should have minimal visible fat marbled through it, and you should trim off any fat around the meat **before** you cook it.

EGGS

Eggs are a good source of protein. They are low in fat, although the yolk is rich in cholesterol. Unless you have a high cholesterol level, you can eat three or four eggs a week. Two eggs make a good serving.

BEANS/LEGUMES

Beans/legumes are excellent as a source of protein and have the added advantage of being low in fat. They make an ideal alternative or addition to meat dishes. They are rich in carbohydrate and fiber, so include them often. Three-quarters of a cup of cooked beans/legumes is a good serving size.

NUTS AND SEEDS

Nuts and seeds—and products made from them, such as peanut butter and tahini—are a valuable source of protein, but are high in fat, so eat them in small amounts.

MILK AND MILK PRODUCTS

Regular milk and dairy products are high in fat, but there are many low-fat products available and you would do well to use them:

- Skim or low-fat milks

- Skim or low-fat yogurts, natural or artificially sweetened

- Skim or low-fat cheeses

- Low-fat ice creams

When choosing low-fat cheeses, preferably choose those with less than 20 percent fat. When choosing low-fat ice creams choose those with less than 4 percent fat. Also try to avoid eating cream and sour cream—save them for special occasions and, even then, use them in small amounts.

Milk as a Carbohydrate Source

Milk and yogurt contain the carbohydrate lactose (milk sugar). One cup of milk or yogurt will give you roughly the same amount of carbohydrate as a slice of bread. The use of small amounts of milk such as that taken in tea or coffee need not be considered as a carbohydrate source. A cup of milk or yogurt makes a good alternative to other carbohydrate foods.

> **A Special Note on Milk**
>
> *Dairy products are important sources of protein and calcium. Women, particularly, should be aware of the value of dairy products in helping protect them from osteoporosis (loss of calcium from bones). Calcium, of course, plays a vital part in good bone health.*
>
> *Adult men should include 1½ cups of milk or the equivalent in dairy products in their daily diet.*
>
> *Children, adolescents, and adult women (including those who are pregnant, breast-feeding or post-menopausal) should include at least four cups of milk or the equivalent in dairy products in their daily diet.*
>
> *The following each contain **about** the **same quantity** of calcium:*
>
> *8 fl oz milk   8 fl oz yogurt   1⅓ oz piece of cheese*

LIMIT THE AMOUNT OF ALCOHOL YOU DRINK

Alcoholic drinks are high in calories, and can contribute to weight gain. They can also react with diabetes tablets or insulin, causing a drop in your blood glucose level. Too much alcohol taken regularly can lead to a rise in the fat level in your blood which increases the risk of heart disease.

Having diabetes does not mean that you cannot drink alcohol at all. It simply means moderation and good sense. **If you drink alcohol, then we recommend that you do not drink more than one or two standard alcoholic drinks a day.** By a "standard" drink we mean a small—a 7 fl oz glass of beer; a 5 fl oz glass of wine; a 1 fl oz shot of spirits such as whisky, vodka, or gin; or a 2 fl oz glass of dry vermouth or dry sherry.

Remember that many drinks such as beer, sweet wines and liqueurs also contain significant amounts of carbohydrate which may increase your blood glucose level. So, it's best to choose a dry rather than a sweet wine, and to drink low-alcohol beer rather than the regular ones.

Don't be lulled into a false sense of security by drinking "lite" or "diet beers." These contain a large amount of alcohol and calories and should be treated as if they were ordinary alcoholic drinks when it comes to quantity.

Here are Some Preferred Choices in Alcoholic Drinks:

Dry wines (riesling, chablis, burgundy, claret, graves); brut champagnes; spirits; low-alcohol beers (2.5 percent or less); dry fortified wines, such as dry vermouth and dry sherry.

A Note About Mixers:

When using mixers, be aware that all the regular soft drinks contain a large amount of refined sugar, and we do not advise their use. But water and low-calorie mixers can be used freely, as follows:

- *Water*
- *Soda water*
- *Unflavored mineral water*
- *Low-calorie drinks including tonic, dry ginger ale, cola-flavored drinks and lemonade.*

Most importantly, don't drink alcohol on an empty stomach. **Always** eat some starchy food when you drink, for example, dry crackers with your whisky, a meal with your wine.

Unsweetened fruit juice and milk contain carbohydrate and are useful as mixers in situations where no better source of carbohydrate is available, such as a slice of bread or a dry cracker.

If you are taking diabetes medication, and you drink alcohol without having carbohydrate, your blood glucose level may drop too low, leading to **hypoglycemia or "hypo" which can be serious and require urgent action**. On page 45 we tell you more about hypoglycemia, how to prevent and treat it.

CONTROL YOUR WEIGHT

Being overweight makes diabetes more difficult to control. The extra body fat alters the cell receptor sites as described on page 5 so that they are unable to accept the combination of insulin and glucose. As a result, blood glucose levels remain too high.

Fortunately, once you lose excess weight, the receptor sites are reactivated, allowing insulin to be taken up effectively so that your blood glucose level can be controlled without medication or with minimal amounts of tablets or injected insulin.

MetLife Height and Weight Table*

Weights for ages 25–59 based on lowest mortality. Weights include indoor clothing weight 3 lbs. for women and 5 lbs. for men. Heights include shoes with 1" heels.

Height	Small Frame	Medium Frame	Large Frame
Men			
5' 2"	128–134	131–141	138–150
5' 3"	130–136	133–143	140–153
5' 4"	132–138	135–145	142–156
5' 5"	134–140	137–148	144–160
5' 6"	136–142	139–151	146–164
5' 7"	138–145	142–154	149–168
5' 8"	140–148	145–157	152–172
5' 9"	142–151	148–160	155–176
5' 10"	144–154	151–163	158–180
5' 11"	146–157	154–166	161–184
6'	149–160	157–170	164–188
6' 1"	152–164	160–174	168–192
6' 2"	155–168	164–178	172–197
6' 3"	158–172	167–182	176–202
6' 4"	162–176	171–187	181–207
Women			
4' 10"	102–111	109–121	118–131
4' 11"	103–113	111–123	120–134
5'	104–115	113–126	122–137
5' 1"	106–118	115–129	125–140
5' 2"	108–121	118–132	128–143
5' 3"	111–124	121–135	131–147
5' 4"	114–127	124–138	134–151
5' 5"	117–130	127–141	137–155
5' 6"	120–133	130–144	140–159
5' 7"	123–136	133–147	143–163
5' 8"	126–139	136–150	146–167
5' 9"	129–142	139–153	149–170
5' 10"	132–145	142–156	152–173
5' 11"	135–148	145–159	155–176
6'	138–151	148–162	158–179

*Courtesy of Metropolitan Life Insurance Company, *Statistical Bulletin*.

If you are overweight, losing weight is the key to good diabetes control, and should be a priority. It will also benefit your overall health. Check the chart on page 23 to see whether you need to maintain or lose weight.

Whether you need to maintain or lose weight, the guidelines given in this book will help you achieve your goal. If you need to lose weight you will have to reduce your calorie intake.

By limiting your fat and sugar intake, and having more foods high in carbohydrate and fiber, you should be able to control your weight and still eat enough to satisfy your appetite.

While you are losing weight, it is important to maintain your health by eating regular meals that supply all your nutritional needs. Avoid crash diets and quick solutions—they offer no long term benefits. Developing a healthy eating pattern over a period of time will help you achieve and maintain a lower weight.

On the Shelves

You will need to become a smart consumer. By knowing what your options are, and by carefully reading the nutrition labels, you will be able to make the right choices. The following information should help guide you through the aisles of your local market.

"DIABETIC" or "CARBOHYDRATE MODIFIED" PRODUCTS

You will find many foods targeted at people with diabetes that fall into two main groups:

High fat—diabetic (carbohydrate modified) chocolates, ice creams, cookies, and crackers.

Low fat—jams, pickles and sauces.

Generally, you will find that these specialized products are more expensive and do not taste as good as the regular variety.

Small amounts of either the regular or specialized alternatives are acceptable; **however those who are overweight should limit their use of the high fat group to an occasional treat.**

LOW-CALORIE PRODUCTS

These products are marketed for people who want to lose weight. They are suitable for people with diabetes and you can use them freely. Here are some of them:

* Low-calorie jams and jelly, low-calorie soft drinks and cordials, low-oil or no-oil salad dressings.

"SUGAR FREE" PRODUCTS

Foods labelled as 'sugar free' are only free of added sugar, and they should not be confused with low-calorie products. Some are high in naturally occurring sugars such as fructose, lactose, grape juice, apple concentrate, and pear juice. The calorie value of these products can be as high as regular sweetened products; you should use them sparingly.

If you are still uncertain whether a product is suitable, read the label carefully and, if it appears high in these sugars, ask your dietitian for advice (see the next section for information on understanding labels).

ARTIFICIAL SWEETENERS

Wherever possible, enjoy the natural sweetness of food. But if you must have added sweetness, you can use the many alternatives to sugar available on the market.

There has been some controversy about the safety of some of these products with prolonged and frequent use. However, these concerns have not been proved and overweight is considered a far greater risk to good health than any of these sweeteners.

Some artificial sweeteners contain calories and others do not, or have very small amounts.

Artificial Sweeteners Which Have Negligible Calories Include:

ACESULFAME - K (Trade name Sunett). 200 times sweeter than sugar, and was approved in the U.S. in 1988. It is marketed as "Sweet One" and "Swiss Sweet."

It is used in a variety of manufactured food products such as fruit drinks and soft drinks, and in sweetened dairy products such as yogurts. It is not available as a table sweetener.

It is not metabolized by the body, therefore does not contribute to calorie intake.

Acesulfame-K is heat-stable, so it is safe for use in cooking and baking.

ASPARTAME. It was discovered by chance when a scientist was researching ulcer drugs. For domestic use it is marketed as "Equal" and we have used it in many of our recipes. Under the trade name "Nutrasweet" it sweetens a host of commercially prepared foods and beverages.

Because it tends to break down under high heat or during lengthy cooking, aspartame is not suitable for cooking, unless you add it at the end of the process. This is not always possible, for instance in baking, and so other sweeteners should be used.

Aspartame is 180 times sweeter than sugar, dissolves in liquid (making it useful as a sweetener in tea and coffee), and has no unpleasant after-taste.

SACCHARIN. The oldest of the artificial sweeteners, it was discovered in 1879 and went into commercial use in the early 1900s. It is 300 times sweeter than sugar; however, up to one in four people notice a bitter or metallic after-taste in foods sweetened with it. Saccharin is soluble and therefore useful as a sweetener; however, it is best added as late as possible in the cooking process to limit the development of any bitter after-taste.

In terms of safety, saccharin has been intensively studied and it would appear that, in the quantities any human is likely to take, it has no dangerous side effects.

Artificial Sweeteners Supplying Calories Include:

SORBITOL. It is manufactured commercially from glucose obtained from natural sources such as fruits. It is absorbed slowly into the bloodstream and, therefore, does not cause a major increase in blood glucose level, although it supplies as many calories as other sugars. Because of the calories it contains, we would recommend that you avoid or limit its use. Be aware, too, that more than 1½ oz of sorbitol taken in a single day may have a laxative effect.

MANNITOL. This is a sugar alcohol made from mannose which is found in seaweed and some other natural products. It is approximately half as sweet as sugar and may have a mild laxative effect if you take more than ½ oz a day. It contributes only about 2 calories per gram because it is poorly absorbed.

FRUCTOSE. Occurring naturally in fruits and honey, it can be purchased as a white powder which is slightly sweeter than sugar, but contains the same amount of calories per weight.

Fructose is absorbed more slowly than sugar, so it does not increase the level of blood glucose as quickly or to the same extent following absorption. It also does not require as much insulin for its use in the body. For these reasons it is sometimes used to sweeten foods for people with diabetes; however, because of its calorie content, and its overall effect on the blood glucose level, we recommend it be used sparingly and, preferably, not at all.

LACTOSE. Lactose or milk sugar is frequently used as a bulking agent to produce powdered artificial sweeteners which resemble sugar in appearance. It contributes the same amount of calories as any other sugars. Use this type of sweetener with caution.

Read the labels of your sweeteners carefully. Many are made from combinations of sweeteners, or are bulked up with agents such as lactose.

TIPS AND TRAPS WHEN USING ARTIFICIAL SWEETENERS

- Artificial sweeteners are much sweeter than sugar, so you only need a small amount.

- Some people's taste buds are very sensitive to these products, and they describe a lingering bitter or metallic after-taste. Using a different sweetener or using less of the product may help you overcome this.

- Saccharin develops a bitter taste when boiled, particularly when cooked with fruit. Always add this sweetener after the fruit has been cooked and has cooled. Where food is not boiled, for example, when baking an egg custard, the sweetener can be added before cooking.

- Aspartame loses it sweetness when heated and is not suitable for dishes which require heating.

- Aspartame loses it sweetness with prolonged storage in liquids. For example, soft drink sweetened with aspartame does not store well.

- Some sweeteners are mixed with other sugars such as lactose and glucose to reduce the concentration of their sweetness, and to enable you to sprinkle them. This adds calories, so use them sparingly.

- Some products are advertised as sugar free, but if you read the label, you will see that they contain quite large amounts of sweeteners such as sorbitol and fructose.

MAKING SENSE OF FOOD LABELS

Many commercial foods that you can buy at the supermarket contain a lot of sugar and/or fat and may be low in fiber, making them unsuitable for you. But how do you know which ones they are?

Reading labels provides valuable information, but is not always as straightforward as it looks. You need to know how to interpret the information so you can make wise choices.

Ingredient List

There are food labelling laws in America which state that all ingredients in a product must appear on the label, listed in order of quantity. This means the ingredient used in the greatest amount is listed first, and that used in the smallest amount is listed last.

For example, let us look at a product label including the following ingredients: **Wheat flour, oats, beef fat, malt extract, raisins, flavoring, salt.**

There is more wheat flour in this product than anything else, and less salt.

To help you decide which products are suitable or unsuitable, we have listed some of the names used for fat, sugar and fiber:

FAT	SUGAR		FIBER
beef fat	apple concentrate	mannitol	bran
beef tallow	brown sugar	molasses	oatbran
butter fat	corn syrup	pear concentrate	ricebran
coconut cream	dextrose	sorbitol	rolled oats
coconut oil	glucose	sucrose	wheat germ
corn oil	fructose	treacle	whole grain
cottonseed oil	golden syrup	xylitol	whole wheat
lard	grape concentrate		
margarine	honey		
oil	invert sugar		
shortening	lactose		
soy bean oil	malt		
vegetable oil	malt extract		
	maltose		

Nutrition Information

All commercially produced foods should include a food label showing nutrient composition. This information is of greater value than the ingredient list as it is more accurate and allows you to make product comparison more easily.

On the new food label, terms once used inconsistently, and often misleadingly, now must be applied uniformly to insure that such terms mean the same thing on each product on which they appear. Following are definitions of some of the most frequently used terms.

- **Free.** The product contains no amount of, or only "physiologically inconsequential" amounts of one or more of these components: fat, saturated fat, cholesterol, sodium, sugars, and calories. For instance, "calorie free" means that there are fewer than 5 calories per serving, and "sugar free" and "fat free" indicate that there are less than 0.5 grams per serving. "Saturated fat free" indicates that there are less than 0.5 grams per serving and the level of trans fatty acids does not exceed 1 percent of total fat.

- **Low.** This food could be eaten frequently without exceeding dietary guidelines for one or more of the following components: fat, saturated fat, cholesterol, sodium, and calories. Thus, the following terms are used:

Low fat. 3 grams or less per serving, and if the serving is 30 grams or less or 2 tablespoons or less, per 50 grams of the food.

Low saturated fat. 1 gram or less per serving and not more than 15 percent of calories from saturated fatty acids.

Low sodium. Less than 140 mgs per serving.

Very low sodium. Less than 35 mgs per serving.

Low cholesterol. Less than 20 mgs per serving.

Low calorie. 40 calories or less per serving.

- **No added sugar, without added sugar, no sugar added.** No sugars added during processing or packing, including ingredients that contain sugars (for example, fruit juices, applesauce, or dried fruit). Processing does not increase the sugar content above the amount naturally present in the ingredients. The food that it resembles and for which it substitutes normally contains added sugars. If the product doesn't meet the requirements for a low- or reduced-calorie food, the product bears a statement saying so and directs consumers' attention to the nutrition panel for further information on sugars and calorie content.

- **Lean and extra lean.** The following terms can be used to describe the fat content of meat, poultry, and seafood:

  Lean. Less than 10 grams of fat, less than 4 grams of saturated fat, and less than 95 mgs of cholesterol per serving and per 100 grams.

  Extra lean. Less than 5 grams of fat, less than 2 grams of saturated fat, and less than 95 mgs of cholesterol per serving and per 100 grams.

- **High.** One serving of the food contains 20% or more of the Daily Value for a particular nutrient.

- **Good source.** One serving of the food contains 10% to 19% of the Daily Value for a particular nutrient.

- **Reduced.** A nutritionally altered product contains 25% less of a nutrient or of calories than the regular, or reference, product.

- **Less.** A food, whether altered or not, contains 25% less of a nutrient or of calories than the reference food.

- **Light.** A nutritionally altered product contains one-third fewer calories or half of the fat of the reference food, or the sodium content of a low-calorie, low-fat food has been reduced by 50%.

- **More.** One serving of the food, altered or not, contains a nutrient in a quantity that is at least 10% of the Daily Value more than the reference food.

Below is an example of a food label.

Serving Size. Similar foods (like cereals, cookies, etc.) have similar serving sizes. Be sure to compare the manufacturer's serving size with what you call a serving.

Total Fat. Compare the fat grams per serving to your personal fat budget to see how the food fits into your diet.

Saturated Fat. This should constitute no more than $\frac{1}{3}$ of your total fat budget. Realize that artery-clogging trans fats are not included in this number, but are part of the total fat figure.

Cholesterol. Limit yourself to 300 milligrams per day.

Sodium. Limit yourself to 2,400 milligrams a day.

Protein. Aim for .36 gram per pound of ideal body weight per day.

Nutrients. Expressed as a percentage of the Daily Value—a recommended daily amount based on a 2,000-calorie diet—this may not reflect your personal requirements.

Nutrition Facts

Serving Size ½ cup (114g)
Servings Per Container 4

Amount Per Serving

Calories 90   Calories from Fat 30

	% Daily Value*
Total Fat 3g	5%
Saturated fat 0g	0%
Cholesterol 0mg	0%
Sodium 300mg	13%
Total Carbohydrate 13g	4%
Dietary Fiber 3g	12%
Sugars 3g	
Protein 3g	

Vitamin A 80% • Vitamin C 60% • Calcium 4% • Iron 4%

*Percent Daily Values are based on a 2,000 calorie diet. Your Daily Values may be higher or lower depending on your calorie needs:

Nutrient		2,000 Calories	2,500 Calories
Total fat	Less than	65g	80g
Sat Fat	Less than	20g	25g
Cholesterol	Less than	300mg	300mg
Sodium	Less than	2,400mg	2,400mg
Total Carbohydrate		300g	375g
Fiber		25g	30g

Calories per gram:
Fat 9 • Carbohydrates 4 • Protein 4

Calories. Compare the calories per serving to your personal calorie budget to see how the food fits into your diet.

Calories From Fat. This figure tells you how many of the calories in the product are contributed by fat. Your diet should get no more than 20% to 25% of its calories from fat. If you stick to your fat budget, this will automatically fall into place.

Dietary Fiber. Aim for at least 25 grams per day.

Sugar. Limit yourself to 50 grams of refined sugar per day. Realize that this number doesn't discriminate between natural, higher-nutrient fruit and milk sugars, and nutrient-poor refined sugars.

Daily Values Percentages and Footnotes. Both the Daily Value footnotes provided at the bottom of the label and the % Daily Value data found higher on the label assume a diet of either 2,000 or 2,500 calories. Also, the Daily Value for fat assumes you want to limit fat to 30% of calorie intake. If you're aiming for fewer calories or less fat, this information will overestimate your needs.

The Nutrition Facts Label at a Glance

BETTER CEREAL CHOICES

Start your day right with cereal for breakfast. With the great number of products available, it is difficult to know which ones to choose. Your best choices are high in fiber and low in added sugar (less than 3 grams).

To help you make a sensible choice, we have listed those we recommend. This may not be a complete list as new products are coming onto the market all the time. For cereals not on the following list, read the labels and use our guidelines.

To be included on our recommended list, 1 ounce of cereal had to contain no more than 5 grams of sugar, and at least 2.5 grams or more of dietary fiber.

Planning Your Meals

We've given you the guidelines, now comes the application. What you choose and the quantity you eat will depend on your energy requirements and your weight, as well as on that very important factor, your preferences.

Recommended Cereal Choices

The following chart lists nutrition information for one ounce of each cereal that is included on our recommended list.

Product	Fat (g)	Fiber (g)	Sugar (g)
General Mills Cheerios	2	3	1
General Mills Fiber One*	1	13	0
General Mills Total or Wheaties+	1	3	3
Kellogg's All-Bran w/Extra Fiber*+	0	14	0
Kellogg's Bran Flakes	0	5	5
Kellogg's Nutri-Grain Wheat	0	3	2
Nabisco Shredded Wheat	1	3	0
Nabisco Shredded Wheat 'n Bran	1	4	0
Post Grape-Nuts	0	3	3
Puffed Kashi	0	3	0
Ralston Whole Grain Wheat Chex+	1	3	3
Weetabix	1	3	2
Wheatena Hot Cereal	1	5	0

* sweetened with aspartame
+ contains BHA or BHT

YOUR ENERGY NEEDS

The following chart shows approximate calorie needs for people of different age, sex, and healthy weight. If you are active your needs may be greater; if you are physically inactive your needs may be less.

For further information or guidance discuss this with your dietitian.

Median Heights and Weights and Recommended Calorie Intake

Subject	Weight (lb)	Height (in)	Resting Energy Expenditure	Active Energy Expenditure
Infants			*(calories per day)*	*(calories per day)*
0–6 mos.	13	24	320	650
6 mos.–1 year	20	28	500	850
Children				
1–3 years	29	35	740	1,300
4–6 years	44	44	950	1,800
7–10 years	62	52	1,130	2,000
Males				
11–14 years	99	62	1,440	2,500
15–18 years	145	69	1,760	3,000
19–24 years	160	70	1,780	2,900
25–50 years	174	70	1,800	2,900
51+ years	170	68	1,530	2,300
Females				
11–14 years	101	62	1,310	2,200
15–18 years	120	64	1,370	2,200
19–24 years	128	65	1,350	2,200
25–50 years	138	64	1,380	2,200
51+ years	143	63	1,280	1,900
Pregnant				
2nd–3rd trimester				+300
Lactating				+500

YOUR CARBOHYDRATE, FAT, AND PROTEIN NEEDS

The average American gets 35 percent of his or her calories from carbohydrate. A healthier percentage is 50–60 percent.

The average intake of calories from protein is 20–30 percent and should be reduced to 15–20 percent, while the fat average of 45–55 percent of calories should be reduced to 30–35 percent.

The following chart gives you the amount of carbohydrate, protein, and fat you need to eat to meet the recommended percentage intake for varying energy levels.

YOUR CARBOHYDRATE, PROTEIN AND FAT REQUIREMENTS

Calories	Carbohydrate 50–60% (g)	Protein 15–20% (g)	Fat 30% (g)
1200	150–165	45–60	40
1350	170–185	50–68	45
1500	190–205	56–75	50
1650	205–230	61–83	55
1800	225–250	67–90	60
1950	245–270	72–98	65
2100	260–290	78–105	70
2250	280–310	83–113	78
2400	300–330	89–120	80

MORE ABOUT CARBOHYDRATE

If you are already managing your diet, you may be doing it by various methods such as simply avoiding too much sugar and fat, or by measuring "servings" of food which contain 15g of carbohydrate ("portions" or "exchanges"). If you are unsure about the size of servings, speak to your dietitian or diabetes educator, who can give you precise portions.

The figures for carbohydrate that you are using may differ from the ones we give, but ours reflect the latest information. If your carbohydrate level is currently low and you increase it, you may find that your blood glucose levels are higher for a short while. Your medication may need adjusting temporarily. Discuss this with your doctor, diabetes educator, or dietitian *before* making drastic dietary changes.

For good control of your blood glucose level, older, inactive people should eat at least three or four servings of high-carbohydrate, high-fiber foods at each of their three daily meals (45-60 grams of carbohydrate per meal).

Younger and/or more active people may need to eat five, six or more carbohydrate servings at each meal (at least 75 grams of carbohydrate per meal).

Remember that the high-carbohydrate, high-fiber foods include bread, cereals, beans/legumes, vegetables and fruits. On page 14 we have shown you approximate serving sizes. Each of the carbohydrate servings shown will give you approximately 15 grams of carbohydrate.

We have also detailed the carbohydrate content of each recipe in this book so you know how much carbohydrate you are eating at each meal. For instance, one serving of Bombay Burgers (page 93) will give you about 20 grams of carbohydrate. When you accompany this with a whole grain roll, a green salad and a serving of fruit, you have an ideal meal containing 3–4 servings (about 60 grams) of carbohydrate. The addition of a bowl of Beef and Bean Soup (page 89) will increase this to five servings (about 75 grams) of carbohydrate.

Of course, your carbohydrate intake can be made up of half servings or double servings, depending on what suits you. Remember, exact proportions of servings is very individualized and depends on many factors. It is important to discuss this with your diabetes educator.

Generally, we do not recommend snacking between meals for older, less active people. If you are young, active or involved in vigorous exercise, or if your medications make it necessary, you may need to include high-carbohydrate snacks in your eating plan. But remember, snacking can contribute unnecessary calories which, in turn, can lead to putting on weight.

On the next page we have a simple meal plan which shows you how to put into practice the information we give. The carbohydrate-rich foods have been **highlighted** for easy identification.

Simple Meal Plan

Breakfast

1 serving **whole grain cereal** with low-fat milk

1 serving **fruit**

1-2 slices **whole wheat toast** or **rye bread** and a thin layer of margarine or low-fat spread

Lunch

2 slices **whole grain rye bread** or **bread roll** and a thin layer of margarine or low-fat spread

1 thin slice of lean red meat or chicken (no skin) or tuna or salmon or egg or low-fat cheese

plenty of salad vegetables

1 serving **fruit**

Dinner

2–3 oz serving lean red or white meat or fish

2 servings **starchy vegetables** or **rice** or **pasta**

plenty of non-starchy vegetables

1 slice **whole grain** or **rye bread** or a **bread roll**

1 serving **fruit** and or low-fat yogurt

Bedtime snack

1 serving **whole grain rye bread** or **whole grain crackers** and/or 1 cup low-fat milk as drink

PLANNING YOUR MEALS

You know your calorie requirements, and how much of each of the nutrients you need daily. You also know that you should spread your carbohydrate intake throughout the day. The following pages show you how to take this information and convert it into food.

TIMING YOUR MEALS

To help you control your blood glucose level, you should eat regular meals.

Sample Meal Plans

Water, tea, coffee, or other low-calorie beverage may be drunk with or between meals as desired.

For 1,200 Calories

Breakfast

⅓ cup Meg's Muesli (page 66)
  with 1 cup skim milk
1 slice whole wheat bread with 1 teaspoon margarine

Lunch

Turkey sandwich with 2 oz turkey, lettuce, tomato, and 1 teaspoon mayonnaise
Apple

Dinner

1 serving Saté Chicken (page 130)
⅔ cup brown rice
Salad with 2 tablespoons Creamy Yogurt Dressing (page 188)
1 cup broccoli with 1 teaspoon margarine
¾ cup fresh fruit salad

Bedtime Snack

1 cup skim milk

For 1,500 Calories

Breakfast

⅓ cup Meg's Muesli (page 66)
  with 1 cup skim milk and ½ banana
1 slice whole wheat bread with 1 teaspoon margarine

Lunch

Turkey sandwich with 2 oz turkey, lettuce, tomato, and 1 teaspoon mayonnaise
Apple
Carrot sticks

Dinner

1 serving Saté Chicken (page 130)
⅔ cup brown rice
Salad with 2 tablespoons Creamy Yogurt Dressing (page 188)
1 cup broccoli with 1 teaspoon margarine
¾ cup fresh fruit salad

Bedtime Snack

6 low-fat whole wheat crackers
  with 1 tablespoon peanut butter
1 cup skim milk

Nutrition Data:	Calories 1192
	Carbohydrate 151g
	Protein 75g
	Fat 32g
% Calories From:	Carbohydrate: 51%
	Protein: 25%
	Fat: 24%
Carb. Distribution:	Breakfast 39g
	Lunch 50g
	Dinner 50g
	Snack 12g

Nutrition Data:	Calories 1505
	Carbohydrate 190g
	Protein 85g
	Fat 45g
% Calories From:	Carbohydrate: 50%
	Protein: 22%
	Fat: 28%
Carb. Distribution:	Breakfast 51g
	Lunch 52g
	Dinner 60g
	Snack 27g

For 1,800 Calories

Breakfast

⅔ cup Meg's Muesli (page 66)
  with 1 cup skim milk
1 slice whole wheat bread with 1 teaspoon
  margarine
½ banana

Lunch

Turkey sandwich with 2 oz turkey, lettuce,
  tomato, and 1 teaspoon mayonnaise
1 ounce pretzels
1 cup unsweetened applesauce

Dinner

Saté Chicken (page 130)
1 cup brown rice
Salad with 2 tablespoons Creamy Yogurt Dressing
  (page 188)
1 cup broccoli with 1 teaspoon margarine
¾ cup fresh fruit salad

Bedtime Snack

6 low-fat whole wheat crackers with
  1 tablespoon peanut butter
1 cup skim milk

For 2,400 Calories

Breakfast

⅔ cup Meg's Muesli (page 66) with 1 cup skim
  milk and whole banana
1 slice whole wheat bread with 2 teaspoons
  margarine
1 poached egg

Lunch

Turkey sandwich with 3 oz turkey, lettuce,
  tomato, and 1 teaspoon mayonnaise
1 ounce pretzels
1 cup unsweetened applesauce
1 cup skim milk

Dinner

6 ounces tomato juice
1 serving Saté Chicken (page 130)
1 cup brown rice
Salad with 2 tablespoons Creamy Yogurt Dressing
  (page 188)
Small whole wheat roll with 2 teaspoons
  margarine
1 cup broccoli
¾ cup fresh fruit salad

Bedtime Snack

Peanut butter sandwich with 2 slices whole wheat
  bread, 2 tablespoons peanut butter, and
  1 tablespoon all fruit jam
1 cup skim milk

Nutrition Data:	Calories 1808
	Carbohydrate 237g
	Protein 98g
	Fat 52g
% Calories From:	Carbohydrate: 52%
	Protein: 22%
	Fat: 26%
Carb. Distribution:	Breakfast 65g
	Lunch 70g
	Dinner 75g
	Snack 27g

Nutrition Data:	Calories 2366
	Carbohydrate 300g
	Protein 130g
	Fat 72g
% Calories From:	Carbohydrate: 51%
	Protein: 22%
	Fat: 27%
Carb. Distribution:	Breakfast 70g
	Lunch 78g
	Dinner 95g
	Snack 57g

Sample Vegetarian Meal Plans

Water, tea, coffee, or other low-calorie beverage may be drunk with or between meals as desired.

For 1,200 Calories

Breakfast
⅓ cup Meg's Muesli (page 66) topped with
  1 cup skim milk
1 slice whole wheat bread with 1 teaspoon
  margarine

Lunch
1 sandwich made with 2 slices pumpernickel
  bread with 2 oz low-fat cheese, lettuce,
  tomato, mustard, 1 teaspoon mayonnaise
Apple

Dinner
1 serving Jumping Bean Bake (page 138)
1 serving Tossed Salad (page 170) with
  2 tablespoons Creamy Yogurt Dressing
  (page 188)

Bedtime Snack
1 cup skim milk

For 1,500 Calories

Breakfast
⅓ cup Meg's Muesli (page 66) topped with
  ½ sliced banana and 1 cup skim milk
1 slice whole wheat bread with 1 teaspoon
  margarine

Lunch
1 sandwich made with 2 slices pumpernickel
  bread with 2 oz low-fat cheese, lettuce,
  tomato, mustard, 1 teaspoon mayonnaise
Apple
Carrot sticks

Dinner
1 serving Jumping Bean Bake (page 138)
1 serving Tossed Salad (page 170) with
  2 tablespoons Creamy Yogurt Dressing
  (page 188)
1 cup broccoli

Bedtime Snack
1 cup skim milk
6 low-fat whole wheat crackers
1 teaspoon peanut butter

Nutrition Data:	Calories 1206
	Carbohydrate 159g
	Protein 78g
	Fat 30g
% Calories From:	Carbohydrate: 52%
	Protein: 25%
	Fat: 23%
Carb. Distribution:	Breakfast 40g
	Lunch 45g
	Dinner 62g
	Snack 12g

Nutrition Data:	Calories 1517
	Carbohydrate 201g
	Protein 86g
	Fat 41g
% Calories From:	Carbohydrate: 53%
	Protein: 23%
	Fat: 24%
Carb. Distribution:	Breakfast 49g
	Lunch 55g
	Dinner 70g
	Snack 27g

For 1,800 Calories

Breakfast

⅓ cup Meg's Muesli (page 66) topped with
  ½ banana and 1 cup skim milk
2 slices whole wheat bread spread with 1 teaspoon
  margarine

Lunch

1 sandwich made with 2 slices pumpernickel
  bread with 2 oz low-fat cheese, lettuce,
  tomato, mustard, 1 teaspoon mayonnaise
1 ounce fat-free potato chips
1 cup unsweetened applesauce

Dinner

1 serving Jumping Bean Bake (page 138)
1 serving Tossed Salad (page 170) with
  2 tablespoons Creamy Yogurt Dressing
  (page 188)
1 cup broccoli with 2 teaspoons margarine
1 cup fresh strawberries

Bedtime Snack

6 low-fat whole wheat crackers with
  1 tablespoon peanut butter
1 cup skim milk

For 2,400 Calories

Breakfast

⅔ cup Meg's Muesli (page 66) topped with
  1 whole banana and 1 cup skim milk
1 slice whole wheat bread spread with 2 teaspoons
  margarine

Lunch

1 sandwich made with 2 slices pumpernickel
  bread with 2 oz low-fat cheese, lettuce,
  tomato, mustard, 1 teaspoon mayonnaise
1 cup lentil or bean soup
1 cup unsweetened applesauce

Dinner

V-8 Juice
1 whole wheat bread roll with 1 teaspoon margarine
1 serving Jumping Bean Bake (page 138)
1 serving Tossed Salad (page 170) with
  2 tablespoons Creamy Yogurt Dressing
  (page 188)
1 cup canned apricots (no added sugar)

Bedtime Snack

Peanut butter sandwich with 2 slices whole wheat
bread, 2 tablespoons peanut butter, 1 tablespoon
all-fruit jam
1 cup skim milk

Nutrition Data:	Calories 1803
	Carbohydrate 250g
	Protein 95g
	Fat 47g
% Calories From:	Carbohydrate: 55%
	Protein: 22%
	Fat: 23%
Carb. Distribution:	Breakfast 58g
	Lunch 78g
	Dinner 87g
	Bedtime snack 27g

Nutrition Data:	Calories 2404
	Carbohydrate 337g
	Protein 120g
	Fat 64g
Energy Ratio:	Carbohydrate: 56%
	Protein: 20%
	Fat: 24%
Carb. Distribution:	Breakfast 79g
	Lunch 90g
	Dinner 113g
	Bedtime snack 55g

Timing Your Meals If You Are Not on Medication

If you are not on medication, in most cases spreading your carbohydrate evenly between 3 meals a day is best. Make sure that you have three to four servings of high-carbohydrate foods per meal, but the punctuality of mealtimes is not as important as it would be if you were on medication. However, specifics should be discussed with your dietitian or diabetes educator. Avoid eating snacks between meals if you are overweight.

Timing Your Meals If You Are on Insulin or Diabetes Medication

If you are on medication, then you need to ask what type and when to take it. These questions are best answered in conjunction with your dietitian or diabetes specialist. Find out about your medication so that you can design an eating plan that allows your carbohydrate to be spread in such a way as to keep your blood glucose level within normal range.

An even spread of carbohydrate between three meals daily is usually best, although some people find it easier to regulate blood glucose levels if they eat a carbohydrate-rich snack between meals.

Injected Insulin and Meals

There are various types of insulin available, classified as short, medium, long-acting, or a combination of these depending on when their activity peaks, and the length of action. Short-acting insulins start to lower your blood glucose level immediately after injection; medium and long-acting insulins may take several hours to begin, and then continue to lower your blood glucose level for several more hours.

The time you eat your carbohydrate should match the activity of your insulin. For instance, if you take a short-acting insulin it is important that you have a carbohydrate-rich meal within 30-40 minutes to prevent hypoglycemia.

If you have a medium or long-acting insulin in the morning, make sure you have a lunch that is rich in carbohydrate. If you have an injection before your evening meal, the carbohydrate content of your meal and/or supper should be high, depending on the type of insulin.

If your mealtime is delayed, you may have to take a small carbohydrate snack to prevent your blood glucose level dropping too low before you have your next meal.

You may find that leaving long gaps between meals, or not eating enough carbohydrate at a meal, may cause your blood glucose level to drop too low (we discuss low blood glucose—hypoglycemia—on page 45). Also important is the need to keep your carbohydrate intake even from day to day to prevent unwanted swings in blood glucose level.

Remember, having diabetes does not affect your need for calories, carbohydrate, protein and fat. It only affects the timing and planning of your meals. On the other hand, your meals and meal pattern must suit your lifestyle, and it may be easier to change the timing and dose of your medication rather than your established eating pattern.

EATING OUT

Having diabetes does not mean you have to miss out on the good things in life, such as eating out. What it does mean is that you need to understand your diabetes and how to manage it so that you can live the way you want to. Armed with this book and a bit of practice, you will build up the necessary confidence.

Finding Your Way Around the Menu

Meals out don't have to be dull and a few simple changes can make the menu offered at most restaurants fit your needs.

The waiter can tell you what ingredients are in dishes if you are unsure.

Because restaurant foods may be high in calories, you would be wise to limit yourself to an appetizer and main course, or to a main course and fruit dessert.

SOUPS: Thickened and creamed soups will give you carbohydrate, but may be high in fats too. Ask the waiter to leave out the cream. Or ask for a clear soup or minestrone.

APPETIZERS: Good choices are vegetable salads, shrimp cocktail, steamed seafood, vegetable platter, and stuffed mushrooms. If your appetizer is cooked, like mushrooms, make sure it isn't fried.

MAIN COURSES: Select small servings of lean chicken, fish, meat, or seafood. Vegetarian and pasta dishes are fine, provided they are not loaded with cream, butter, or cheese. To accompany your main course choose pasta, potato, or rice to give you plenty of carbohydrate, and other vegetables and salads to add variety, flavor and color.

BREAD: If the meal you choose does not contain enough carbohydrate, ask for extra bread.

DESSERTS: These are often high-fat, and may contain more sugar than is desirable. If having something sweet to end a meal is important for you, ask for fruit, a simple fruit dessert, a crême caramel or hot soufflé served without cream or rich sauces.

BEVERAGES: Limit your alcohol intake and don't be afraid to ask for a jug of iced water or soda water.

Ethnic Restaurants

Many ethnic restaurants offer good choices. The following ideas may get you started.

Italian: Minestrone soup; pasta with a seafood or tomato sauce; plain salad; crusty bread; and fruit platter.

Chinese: Wonton soup; combination of seafood or meat and vegetables or whole fish in ginger; steamed vegetables; and steamed rice.

Greek: Dolmades; souvlaki; tabbouleh or green salad without dressing; plain pita bread.

Mexican: Taco or burritos; green salad with salsa; refried beans; plain tortillas.

Indian: Tandoori chicken or fish; raita; vegetable curry; chappatis; plain rice.

Take-Out Meals

These are often high in fat and salt. The following are better choices in terms of fat:

- Sandwiches, rolls, or filled pita bread, hamburger (plain meat with lettuce and tomato), souvlaki, barbecued or grilled chicken (no skin), steamed dim sum, baked potatoes (without the sour cream).

Where possible, order a fresh salad or some fruit to balance the meal.

Treats and Special Occasions

Christmas, birthdays and other family get-togethers are especially tempting. If you are the host, choose special recipes from this book for just such occasions. If you are a guest, have a little of the dishes you like, but balance this with vegetables, salad, bread and fruit.

A splurge now and then, on special occasions, does no harm; it's what you do for the rest of the time that counts. Return to your usual eating pattern the next meal. Frequent splurging will contribute to weight gain and poorly controlled diabetes.

TRAVEL

When travelling short distances, try to have your meals at the normal times. When travelling by car, carry crackers, fresh or dried fruits to eat if there are delays.

Overseas travel may mean a change in your normal eating pattern, particularly when you travel quickly across time zones. It is advisable to notify the airline well in advance and request additional fresh fruit, breads, sandwiches and crackers.

If you are going to cross time zones, discuss your insulin and food requirements with your doctor, dietitian or diabetes educator before you leave on the trip.

When travelling in different countries, you can always find suitable food even if it is limited in variety.

SHIFT WORK/ROTATING HOURS

If you are a shift worker, the timing of your meals and medications may vary with the timing of your shifts. Because of the great variation in shifts and individual needs, it is difficult to give suggestions other than strongly advise you to see a dietitian or diabetes educator for help.

Basically you should aim to spread your meals and diabetes medication throughout your waking hours, just as you would on day shift—and treat the day as night. Make sure, if you take your medication prior to going to bed, that you have also eaten.

Special Needs

HYPOGLYCEMIA

When your blood glucose level drops too low, this is known as hypoglycemia. Hypoglycemia is defined as a blood glucose level that falls below the normal range (60–100 mg/dL, or expressed in SI units, 3.33–5.55 mmol/L), which can happen to you if you are on insulin or diabetes tablets. *It does not happen if you are being treated by diet alone.*

How to Recognize Hypoglycemia

The symptoms set in quickly. You may experience **one** or **more** of the following:

- Headache
- Dizziness, vagueness
- Extreme hunger
- Blurred vision
- Drowsiness

- Sweating
- Pins and needles around the mouth
- Paleness, trembling, shaking
- Behavior changes or mood swings (such as bad temper, crying, aggressiveness)

These signs tell you that your blood glucose level may have dropped too low.

Some people who test their blood glucose level regularly may find that their level drops too low without experiencing any symptoms. **If your blood glucose level drops below the normal range, it should be treated as hypoglycemia whether you have symptoms or not.**

What You Should Do

Step 1. **Immediately** take sugar to raise your blood glucose level. Any form of sugar will do but the following are recommended as they are quickly absorbed.
- A regular soft drink or Gatorade—one glass
- Candy such as jelly beans, jubes and life savers—4-5 pieces

- Sugar in water—about three teaspoons in a cup of water

- Glucose, powder or tablets—three teaspoons or 2 tablets

- Honey or jam—about one tablespoon

Do not use low-calorie soft drinks to treat hypoglycemia.

Step 2.   If the symptoms don't improve in five minutes, or become worse, take more sugar as above.

Step 3.   If still no improvement in 10 minutes, **contact your doctor or local hospital without delay.**

Step 4.   **Always follow the concentrated sugar with a snack of more complex carbohydrate** such as fruit, bread, milk, or crackers, or have your next meal if it is due. This will help prevent your blood glucose level from falling again.

   Note: **Do not** count any extra food taken to treat hypoglycemia as part of your regular meal plan. Continue with your usual meals.

If not treated **promptly** and **properly**, hypoglycemia can worsen and lead to unconsciousness. If this happens, others (family, friends, work mates) need to know what to do:

- Roll the person onto his or her left side. Make sure the airway is clear, tilt the chin up and check that the tongue hasn't rolled back.

- Call a doctor or ambulance immediately.

- **Never** give an unconscious person anything to eat or drink.

Medical Treatment

The doctor will usually give an injection of a hormone called glucagon which stimulates the liver to release glucose into the bloodstream. Alternatively, he or she may inject a special glucose solution directly into the vein.

It is advisable to carry a small card containing the above information to assist others should you suffer a "hypo" and become unconscious.

Why It Happens

- Taking too much insulin

- A meal delayed too long

- Not enough carbohydrate in your food

- Extra activity (without having extra carbohydrate foods to supply the extra energy—exercise uses your blood glucose supplies)

- Excess alcohol without carbohydrate—such as drinking whisky on an empty stomach

Simple Precautions to Prevent Hypoglycemia

- Check your food intake to make sure you are having enough carbohydrate with each meal. If meals are delayed, have some carbohydrate in the form of a snack to tide you over.
- Check your dose of insulin or tablets carefully. Taking too much can make your blood glucose level fall too low.
- If you are more active than usual, you may need extra carbohydrate before, during and after the activity, (see Exercise, Sports, and Diabetes, page 56).
- If you are drinking alcohol, make sure you eat food containing carbohydrate with it.

Important: If you are having "hypos" often, consult your doctor to discuss possible causes and solutions. If your diabetes is well controlled, you shouldn't have frequent "hypos."

WHAT TO DO IF YOU ARE ILL

If your diabetes is controlled without medication, don't worry if you are unable to eat properly for a day or two. Eat and drink as desired. If you are unwell for longer than this, discuss it with your doctor.

If you are on insulin or diabetes tablets, you must continue with your medication as usual, **no matter how awful you are feeling.** One of the side effects of various illnesses is that your blood glucose level rises, so your medications are absolutely vital to control this. Equally importantly, you must keep on taking carbohydrate even if you are off your food. To do this, try light meals, drinks high in carbohydrate (we've given a number of suitable recipes) or high-carbohydrate snacks. You may find it easier to have a snack or drink every hour, rather than attempt your usual daily meal pattern.

If you are ill for more than two days, or if your blood glucose is consistently higher than 300 mg/dL, contact your doctor.

The following are easy sources of carbohydrate if you are on medication:

- Homemade or canned soup with toast or dry crackers
- Regular jelly
- Dry crackers
- Plain cookies or cake
- Dry crackers with thinly sliced cheese or tomato
- Ice cream
- Lemonade, ginger ale or other soft drink

- Plain boiled rice, pasta, or noodles
- Toast or sandwich
- Stewed or canned fruit
- Milk drinks such as Ovaltine Lite
- Fruit juice

If nauseous or vomiting, try sipping drinks such as dry ginger ale or lemonade, Gatorade, or dry ginger ale or lemonade with ice cream or milk.

Once you can tolerate any of the above, nibble on a dry cracker or toast, sip chicken noodle soup or try grated apple mixed with a little orange juice.

Vomiting or Diarrhea

If you are vomiting or suffering from diarrhea, be aware that it can lead to dehydration and uncontrolled diabetes. You need urgent treatment so contact your doctor right away.

HIGH BLOOD PRESSURE

Many people with high blood pressure can bring it down by limiting the amount of salt (sodium) in their diet. If overweight, try to reduce your weight as another means of controlling your blood pressure.

If you have high blood pressure you would be wise to:

- Limit the amount of salt you use in cooking
- Avoid adding salt at the table
- Limit the amount of highly salted processed food you eat.

A Note About Salt

We have used a little salt where necessary in our recipes. Some dishes simply taste too bland and unappealing without it. However, we suggest that you always check the flavor of your food before adding salt. Also, remember that in about three weeks you can train your taste buds to appreciate food with less salt, simply by cutting back on the amount of salt you normally eat.

Here is a list of some of the flavoring agents and processed foods that are high in salt:

- Rock, flavored, and vegetable salts—all of them are salt, no matter what the name
- Monosodium glutamate (MSG), flavor boosters, meat and vegetable extracts, broth, stock cubes, stock powders, and packet soups
- Salted, smoked, cured, or pickled meat and fish
- Condiments (sauces), pickles, chutneys, relishes, and dressings
- Canned meat, fish, and vegetables
- Salted snacks, including potato and corn crisps, nuts, and salted crackers
- Take-out foods such as pizza, barbecued chicken
- Cheese

Salt substitutes replace all or part of the sodium chloride with potassium chloride. Although this is a satisfactory substitute for ordinary salt, we would prefer you to train your taste buds to enjoy low-salt foods. It is wise to check with your doctor before using these substitutes.

There are many commercial products which are salt-reduced, such as low-salt breads, crackers, margarines, butters, sauces, canned fish, and vegetables. Use them in place of the regular products and learn to read labels. Look out for the words sodium and salt, and for monosodium glutamate.

Another way in which to give your food zest without using added salt is through herbs and spices. Try adding lemon juice, tomato, onion, garlic, or vinegar for extra flavor.

IF YOU HAVE HIGH BLOOD FAT LEVELS (CHOLESTEROL AND TRIGLYCERIDES)

People who have high blood fat levels have an increased risk of heart and blood vessel disease. You run this risk regardless of whether you are overweight or normal weight. The blood fats of concern are cholesterol and triglycerides. Both of these fats are made in the body as well as provided in foods.

Dietary fats include cholesterol and triglycerides.

Cholesterol is found only in animal products, while triglycerides are found in both animal and vegetable foods.

Foods high in cholesterol include egg yolk, brains, liver, fatty cuts of meat, prawns, squid, fish roe, and dairy foods such as cream, butter and cheese.

95 percent of fat in the diet is in the form of triglycerides. These fats can be categorized as saturated, monounsaturated, or polyunsaturated according to their chemical structure. Animal fats are high in saturated fats which may cause a rise in blood fats and contribute to heart disease. Vegetable fats/oils tend to be higher in monounsaturated and polyunsaturated fats which protect against heart disease.

Fats that are highly saturated include those in meats and dairy foods, and the vegetable fats in cocoa butter and coconut.

Fats which are highly unsaturated (monounsaturated or polyunsaturated) include those in seeds, nuts, olives and avocado or oils made from these foods.

A Note on Saturated Vegetable Fats

Be aware that many commercial foods and fast foods contain vegetable fats that have been hydrogenated. This process changes the fats to saturated fats. It is wise to read labels where possible and to limit the use of commercially prepared high fat and fried foods.

Polyunsaturated and monounsaturated oils and margarines are still high in fats, so they should be used sparingly, particularly if you are overweight.

Although an intake of foods high in fat may increase triglyceride levels, this level can also be raised by alcohol and by eating excessive amounts of refined carbohydrate. High triglyceride levels may also be found in overweight people and in people with undiagnosed or poorly controlled diabetes.

Weight loss and establishing good control of diabetes will help reduce these levels.

Take very seriously our constant reminder to cut down on all fats. Generally, limit all fats and, in particular, animal fats in your diet. See page 18 for Hints to Help You Use Less Fat.

If you are concerned about the amount of fat in your diet or require greater detail on the types of fats, consult a dietitian or contact your local chapter of the American Heart Association.

PREGNANCY AND DIABETES

Diabetes should not stand in the way of a normal, healthy pregnancy. If you have diabetes, make sure that it is under good control where possible before you become pregnant.

You will find that both your nutritional needs and your insulin dosage may need changing while you are pregnant. Get expert help from a dietitian and diabetes specialist and have your diabetes reviewed frequently during your pregnancy so your baby gets the best possible start and you maintain your health throughout.

You may also need to change the timing of your carbohydrate intake at this time, to help with management of your diabetes. It is particularly important that you eat regular meals, especially breakfast and a bedtime snack. Long periods without food may increase your risk of ketosis which can be harmful to you and to your baby.

Developing Diabetes While Pregnant (Gestational Diabetes)

Some women develop diabetes for the first time during pregnancy, usually after the 26th week. Once the baby is born, the symptoms may disappear, and reappear in later pregnancies. Approximately 50 percent of women who develop gestational diabetes go on to develop diabetes again in later life.

To ensure that you and your baby are healthy, once you have been diagnosed as having diabetes, you must take particular care of your diet throughout the remainder of your pregnancy. This is usually all that is needed to control your blood glucose level.

Furthermore, if you control your weight from then on, and make sure your diet is low in fats and added sugars, while high in complex carbohydrate and fiber, you can help prevent or delay the onset of diabetes in later life. This underscores an important point: good nutrition and keeping slim are two of your best defenses against developing diabetes.

CHILDREN AND ADOLESCENTS

You will find the guidelines set out in this book will ensure that children and adolescents with diabetes enjoy the benefits of up-to-date dietary management.

Just as their insulin requirements will vary, so will their dietary needs; it is a good idea to have your child or adolescent's diet reviewed at least annually by a dietitian, and their diabetes and general health monitored regularly. However, do remember that for children and adolescents, food has important social implications. While instilling in your child or adolescent enjoyment of a healthy eating plan, you may have to compromise at times. Food and eating should not become a battlefield, a focus of rebellion, or a source of family tension. To begin with, the entire family would benefit by eating in exactly the same way. This takes away any sense of 'being different' or being deprived.

There is a common misconception that the food you should prepare for your offspring with diabetes is by its very nature unpalatable and "unusual." The meal plans and recipes in this book show just how unnecessary and wrong this view is; teach all your children about a varied and balanced eating plan, encourage a liking for cereals, vegetables and fruit, and you will have achieved something of lifelong value.

Be flexible and make an effort in the kitchen to prepare food that delights and satisfies. Remember, too, that children and adolescents like snacks, so prepare healthy and delicious ones in advance so that you don't hear the complaint "There's nothing to eat," meaning "There is nothing ready prepared that I can pick up in my fingers right away." This avoids problems where children and adolescents turn to fast foods and processed products because they are so easy to get hold of. Providing alternatives is half the battle; good sense will see you through the rest.

TIPS AND TRAPS FOR CHILDREN AND ADOLESCENTS

- With young children, it is important that they take an active part in their diabetes management, including blood glucose monitoring, insulin injections, food choices and planning meals. You will find that the more involved your child is, the less tension is likely to arise.

- Avoid making diabetes the focus of family life; it's just one aspect. Don't force children to eat; you don't always feel hungry, neither do they. Forcing a reluctant child to eat leads to resentment, rebellion and anxiety for everyone. It's totally counter-productive. You may find, in the name of cooperation and family well-being, that you have to sometimes make a temporary compromise on diabetes control for the sake of long-term outcome.

- By learning to monitor his or her own blood glucose level, your child will soon learn the effects different foods have on it.

- Teach your children the benefits of regular meals and a healthy way of eating. It's an investment in their future health. Use this approach and children will come to see healthy eating as a positive aspect of life rather than as a negative aspect of having diabetes. Children (and adults for that matter) should learn that diabetes does not mean being punished or deprived of food.

- It's easy to fall into the trap of replacing uneaten vegetables and cereals with sugary foods because of a fear of hypoglycemia. Children are smart and they will soon learn to manipulate; they may start refusing their meals knowing you may offer them a sweet treat instead. Try offering healthier alternatives in this situation: fruit, milk, or dry crackers will do the trick.

- Encourage your child to carry extra snacks, especially when they will be away from home for long periods such as sleeping out on weekends or going to after-school activities.

- Make sure parents of friends and teachers at school know that your child has diabetes and that they know how to cope with hypoglycemia and sickness.

- Let your child know that there are other children with diabetes. They are neither alone nor unique. Diabetes camps are an excellent way to reduce any sense of isolation. For details on these camps, get in touch with the American Diabetes Association or the local children's hospital.

- Diabetes is not a barrier to normal childhood activities such as parties, sport, staying at friends', trips or school camps, and you should encourage your child to take part.

- The better your child understands his or her diabetes, the more responsibility he or she will take for it and so he or she will cope better with their own changing needs as he or she grows older.

- Don't turn your child into a "closet eater" or "food sneak" by never allowing sweet foods. That old phrase, "moderation in all things" holds good. You may well find that denying your child any sweet foods leads to secret eating and binges. Simply don't make a fuss about fatty or sweet foods; remember that the occasional splurge will not cause any long-term harm.

- Adolescence brings its own special needs. The teen years are a time of exploration, testing and a desire or need for independence. This applies to the issue of food just as much as it does to other realms of behavior. If your teenager has a good knowledge of diabetes management, he or she will know how to be flexible in terms of mealtimes, foods eaten, the amount of insulin needed, and when it is needed. This may cause you considerable anxiety, but you must learn to encourage your children's sense of independence; allow them to learn by their own mistakes.

- For adolescents, the peer pressure to drink alcohol may be strong. While all adolescents should be encouraged not to drink, make sure your teen understands how vital it is to have plenty of carbohydrate if he or she drinks alcohol.

- Adolescents also need to realize **how vital it is to seek medical help the moment they do not feel well.** Failure to do this is a common cause of hospital admissions for uncontrolled diabetes.

- Hormonal changes and growth spurts during adolescence may upset your adolescent's diabetes control even though he or she is doing the right thing. It may be that the whole management routine needs a fresh appraisal.

VEGETARIANS WITH DIABETES

The guidelines in this book are ideal for people who are vegetarian. Many of the recipes have been created with vegetarians in mind, and on pages 39–40 you will find vegetarian meal plans showing how to balance your nutritional needs.

You can follow a vegetarian diet, be well nourished and keep your diabetes under control. But you should also be aware that as a vegetarian you can miss out on some nutrients. It is therefore vital that you know how to plan your diet to ensure these are included in adequate amounts.

To begin with, we suggest that you include dairy products and eggs in your vegetarian eating plan (in other words, what is termed "lacto-ovo vegetarian"). However, if you choose out of matters of conscience or religion to follow a strict vegan lifestyle (in other words, do not eat any animal products at all), we strongly recommend that you consult a dietitian, who will help you plan an adequate diet.

The principles in this book apply to vegetarians; however there are other tips which are particularly important.

TIPS AND TRAPS FOR VEGETARIANS

- The nutrients that may be lacking in a poorly planned diet are: iron, zinc, protein, calcium, cyanocobalamin (vitamin B_{12}), and riboflavin (B_2).

- The best sources of iron and zinc for vegetarians are beans/legumes, whole grain cereal products, green leafy vegetables, and eggs. However, these foods do not release their minerals into your system as readily as do animal sources, such as meat.

- To increase your absorption of iron from non-meat sources, include foods with vitamin C at the same meal. For instance, include citrus fruits, pineapple, tomatoes, or juice made from them when you eat iron-rich food such as cereal products or spinach.

- The tannin in tea interferes with the absorption of iron into your body, so don't finish your meal with a cup of tea.

- Fiber slows the absorption of vitamins and minerals in your digestive tract, so you may have to eat more of certain foods to counter this.

- Eat the recommended daily amounts of dairy products and eggs set out below to ensure your protein, calcium, cyanocobalamin (B_{12}), and riboflavin (B_2) needs are met.

A Guide to Recommended Daily Food Intake for Lacto-Ovo Vegetarians

Milk and dairy products

3 cups milk or the equivalent in cheese and/or yogurt

1 cup milk = $1\frac{1}{3}$ oz hard cheese

= 1 cup yogurt

Note: Low-fat cheeses such as cottage and ricotta are poor sources of calcium.

Other protein-rich foods

We recommend that you eat two servings of the following every day:

- eggs
- beans/legumes
- nuts
- soy bean curd (tofu)

- 1 serving = 2
- 1 serving = 3/4 cup
- 1 serving = 3 oz
- 1 serving = 1 cup (7 oz)

Note: Because vegetarian diets are generally low in high cholesterol foods, don't worry about limiting your intake of eggs.

Guidelines for other foods

Make sure that your daily diet also includes:

Fruits	At least two to three servings
Vegetables	At least five servings
Bread and cereals	A minimum of four servings or more, according to appetite
Fats	1-2 tablespoons, including some table margarine

TIPS FOR VEGANS

- Suitable protein sources include **fortified soy milk**, beans/legumes, nuts, seeds, and cereal products. As the protein quality from these sources is not as good as animal sources, you need to eat a variety of these products every day.

- Alternative cyanocobalamin (B_{12}) sources include **fortified soy milk** (check the label). As only a few milks are fortified, a supplement is recommended.

- Alternative calcium sources include **fortified soy milk** (check the label). Sesame and sunflower seeds, tahini, and almonds contain small amounts of calcium.

- Alternative riboflavin (B2) sources include **fortified soy milk** (check the label), dried fruits, beans/legumes, nuts, and green leafy vegetables.

A Note About Soy Milk and Diabetes

Many brands of soy milk have added sugar (usually in the form of sucrose). This is also common in flavored soy milk, so we advise you to read the labels. Regular soy milks are poor sources of calcium, riboflavin (B_2) and cyanocobalamin (B_{12}).

EXERCISE, SPORTS, AND DIABETES

Regular exercise is important for everyone who wants to achieve and maintain good health. This means at least 30 minutes three times a week. Good forms of exercise include brisk walking, swimming, bike riding, and aerobics. To know whether your body is benefiting from exercise, check your pulse immediately afterwards; it should be faster than your usual resting level.

For people with diabetes, exercise has another function: it helps people with diabetes keep their blood glucose level within normal range. People with **non-insulin dependent diabetes** can improve the control of their diabetes and minimize their need for medication by exercising or playing sports regularly.

If you have insulin-dependent diabetes, regular exercise is important, but requires more careful planning. You will learn from experience how your body reacts to exercise and how best to balance your energy expenditure with the needs of your diabetes.

TIPS AND TRAPS FOR EXERCISE

Hypoglycemia is the most common concern for people on diabetes medication who exercise regularly. However, there are some simple steps you can take to help prevent this problem.

- Where possible, check your blood glucose level before you exercise, especially if you are new to diabetes. If you feel your level is low, then take a carbohydrate snack before you begin exercising. You may find it useful to take another test after the exercise, or during it if it is prolonged, so you become familiar with the effect exercise has on your blood glucose level.

- If you are exercising away from home, make sure you have some carbohydrate foods with you, such as fruit, fruit juice, dried fruit or crackers.

- If you have been doing vigorous exercise, your blood glucose level may continue to drop after you stop exercising, so you should eat some carbohydrate afterwards, too.

- Be aware of dehydration. But don't confuse this with hypoglycemia which relates not to fluids but to blood glucose level. If you exercise vigorously and especially in hot weather, **keep drinking plenty of fluids before, during and after you exercise.**

- When your exercise session is over, quench your thirst with a non-alcoholic drink. Alcohol may lower your blood glucose level further and also has a dehydrating effect.

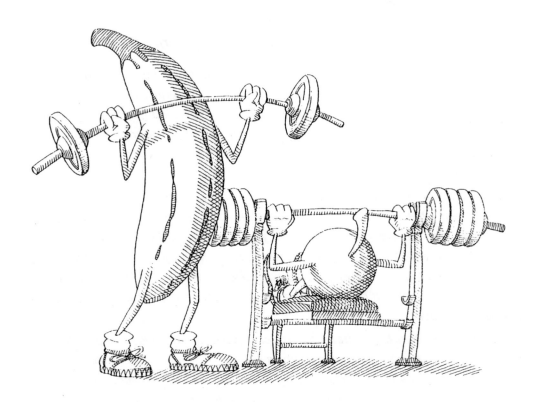

EXERCISE AND YOUR BLOOD GLUCOSE LEVEL
For the person without diabetes

The body is able to keep blood glucose level constant during sport through the release of insulin and other hormones.

When exercise begins, the body normally stops releasing insulin and produces the hormones adrenalin and glucagon which stimulate the liver to release glucose into the blood. The insulin already present in the bloodstream allows the exercising muscles to take up the glucose, converting it to energy and keeping the blood glucose level constant.

As the exercise continues, the blood glucose level normally goes up and the liver then stops releasing glucose. Now the body releases insulin again, so that more glucose can pass into the exercising muscle. This complex mechanism ensures that the blood glucose level normally remains constant.

What happens if you have insulin-dependent diabetes?

If you have insulin-dependent diabetes, you don't have the benefit of this natural control. Once you have taken your insulin injection, you cannot regulate its action. This means that you may have a wide variation in your blood glucose level during and after exercise. However, if you have enough insulin in your system and your blood glucose level is within the normal range at the start of exercise, then you can safely exercise.

If you don't have enough insulin available in your system when you begin exercising—in other words, your blood glucose level is high—your body can misread the situation and release more glucose into your bloodstream from the liver. Because you don't have enough insulin, the glucose can't pass into your muscle cells. As a result, your blood glucose level will rise excessively (hyperglycemia). So check your glucose levels before you begin. You shouldn't exercise if your blood glucose is above 16 mmol/l.

If, on the other hand, you have too much insulin in your blood and your blood glucose level is low, your liver shuts down its release of glucose. The insulin continues to carry glucose to your muscles, leading to a rapid fall in your blood glucose level (hypoglycemia). In this case take more carbohydrate before you begin to exercise.

- Serious athletes with diabetes (and there are many) ensure that their diabetes is well controlled before they begin training. Training is the time to fine tune control. They know that this will ensure peak performance during competition.

How to Adjust Your Food Intake

Once your diabetes is controlled, you will need to learn how to manipulate the balance between food, insulin and activity. The only way to do this properly is to monitor your blood glucose level before, during and after you exercise and experiment until you are confident about the combination which suits your needs best.

Use these recommendations as a starting point to work out your carbohydrate intake and adjust it to suit your individual needs.

Activity	Time	Blood Glucose Level Prior to Activity (mg/dL)	Recommended Additional Carbohydrate Intake
Low Level	½ hour	<100	15g carbohydrates (one serving fruit, bread, crackers, yogurt, or milk).
		>100	No extra food.
Moderate Intensity	1 hour	<100	20–30g carbohydrates (1½–2 servings fruit, bread, crackers, yogurt, and/or milk).
		100–180	15g carbohydrates (one serving fruit, bread, crackers, yogurt, or milk).
		180–300	No extra food (in most cases).
		>300	No extra food. Exercise not recommended: blood glucose level may go up.
Strenuous Activity	1–2 hours	100	45–60g carbohydrates (1 sandwich and fruit and/or milk or yogurt).
		100–180	25–50g carbohydrates (1 sandwich and/or fruit, milk, or yogurt).
		180–300	15g carbohydrates (1 serving fruit, bread, crackers, yogurt, or milk).
		>300	Exercise not recommended: blood glucose level may go up.
Varying Intensity	Long Duration ½–1 day		Insulin may best be decreased. (Conservatively decrease the insulin dose due to peak at time of activity by 10%. A 50% reduction is not uncommon.)
			Increase carbohydrates before, during, and after activity.
			15–50g carbohydrate per hour, such as diluted fruit juice or sports drinks.

How to Modify Recipes

Some of your old favorite family recipes may seem unsuitable if you have diabetes. Before putting them away, see if you can alter them to suit your new eating pattern. You may be able to reduce the fat and sugar, and increase the fiber, without changing the flavor or appearance of the dish very much, if at all.

We have taken an old-fashioned dessert to show you how to adapt it. *The changes in ingredients and method are shown in italics.*

Bread Pudding

4 thin slices bread	*Use whole wheat bread*
4 tbsp sugar	*Use an alternative sweetener or 1 tbsp sugar and vanilla extract for more flavor*
½ cup raisins	
2 tbsp butter	*3 tsp should be enough and use polyunsaturated margarine*
2 eggs	
1 pt milk	*Use low-fat milk*

1. Grease a pie dish.

    Use a non-stick cooking spray.

2. Spread the bread with butter (*margarine*) and layer it in the dish with sugar and raisins sprinkled in between.

    Use far less sugar, or if you prefer a sweet pudding, add sweetener to the eggs and milk.

3. Beat the eggs and milk.

    Add sweetener and vanilla if preferred to sugar.

4. Pour egg mixture over the bread and leave to stand for 10 minutes. Then bake in the oven until the custard is set, approximately 20-25 minutes.

TIPS AND TRAPS IN MODIFYING RECIPES

Main Dishes

- Consider whether you can cut down on the amount of meat. 4 ounces of raw meat per person is sufficient. This means 1 pound should feed four.

- Choose lean cuts and trim off any visible fat.

- If bacon is used as a flavoring, try using a little lean ham, ham bone, or bacon stock cube instead—in which case you will not need to add more salt.

- Reduce fats. For browning foods, use a non-stick pan over high heat to dry-fry foods such as meat. Alternatively, use a cooking spray or a pastry brush to brush a thin layer of oil on the base of the pan—you really need very little to do the trick.

- Don't use more than 2 teaspoons of added fat for a recipe serving four, or leave out the fat if you can.

- If a recipe uses cream or sour cream as a sauce, you can often use non-fat yogurt instead, but remember to add it at the last minute and not allow the sauce to reboil or the yogurt will curdle.

- For white sauces, use low-fat or skim milk in place of regular milk. Use the minimum amount of butter or margarine, or use cornstarch with low-fat milk and don't use fat at all. (Evaporated skim milk can also be used.)

- To add fiber and decrease the meat, include some dried beans or lentils in mixed dishes with meat. This works wonderfully in pasta sauces, lasagne, curries, and casseroles.

Desserts and Cakes

Many of these recipes modify well, so try your old standbys with a few changes, such as:

- Substitute whole wheat flour for white, or, if the result is too heavy, use a half-and-half mixture.

- If you substitute or use whole wheat pastry flour in a recipe, you usually have to add a little more liquid to get a moist result.

- Substitute skim or low-fat milk for regular milk.

- Reduce or remove the butter or margarine. Where a recipe specifies that you cream butter and sugar, minimize the sugar, reduce the butter and rub into the dry ingredients.

- Where you have reduced butter and sugar in a recipe, it will not rise as high, and the texture will be a little denser. Try using a smaller baking tin.

And If Your Recipe Can't Be Modified . . .

Some recipes simply don't look and taste the same if modified. Put these on your list of occasional dishes and keep them as treats—and then only have a small serving.

Pleasures of the Table

USING THE RECIPES IN THIS BOOK

Most of the recipes in this book are simple and quick to prepare. In most cases, we avoid using unusual ingredients, although we slip some in now and again to encourage you to experiment.

Flavor

You can increase or decrease the flavor intensity of recipes to suit your own taste. Experiment with herbs and spices; cut back or add more as you like. Such flavor enhancers will not alter the nutritional value of your food.

If microwaving any of the dishes, you may need to increase the amount of herbs and spices we recommend because microwaving does not always allow for the flavors to develop and combine.

Salt

We follow the good health guideline of "cut back on salt." However, we use common sense, and where we feel that a recipe needs a little salt we add it or use soy sauce or stock cubes. To flavor your food without salt, you might consider using some lemon juice or flavor-enhancing seasonings.

We encourage you to minimize or omit salt wherever possible. Where we refer to soy sauce in the recipes, we suggest you use light or salt-reduced soy sauce.

Sugar

We use a variety of sweetening agents in our recipes, including sugar in small amounts. There are good reasons for this. First, we now know that a small amount of sugar taken in a mixed meal or recipe does not cause a significant rise in the blood glucose level. Second, some recipes, especially baked products, rely on sugar to produce good results. Third, there are some instances where the flavor of sugar is superior to that of artificial sweeteners—it does not alter or lose taste during the cooking process.

You will also see that we use natural sweetening agents other than sucrose (table sugar), such as fruit juice, dried fruits, and fruit juice concentrates, with delicious results. A range of artificial sweeteners are also used.

Fat

We use a number of ways to reduce the fat content of our recipes. For example, we frequently sauté using water or a hot dry pan instead of oil. Where oil is used we have kept it to a minimum by recommending that you brush the frying pan with oil rather than pouring it in.

Generally we use skim or low-fat milk (1.5–2% fat). Likewise, with yogurt; in most cases, you can substitute low-fat natural yogurt for full cream yogurt. But not always: for instance, full-cream yogurt is absolutely necessary in Quick Whole Wheat Bread (page 222).

Where we use cottage cheese, it is always the skim milk variety; ricotta cheese is always low-fat ricotta; low-fat block cheese is cheese of less than 17% fat. Low-fat cream cheese is a mixture of approximately half cottage cheese and half cream cheese where you mix your own, or the commercial variety of less than 17% fat. To enhance the flavor of some recipes, we include a small amount of higher-fat tasty cheeses, such as Parmesan. Here, we use the principle that a small amount goes a long way.

Fiber

We use whole wheat products as much as possible. However, there are times when the texture or flavor of the dish is better with a mixture of whole wheat and refined flours or cereals. In a few recipes, we use the refined product only to give a more traditional result. Using whole wheat flour products gives a heavier or denser texture than white flour, and requires more liquid during cooking. We allow for this in our recipes.

When Using the Oven

Always turn your oven on in plenty of time so it is at the correct temperature when you are ready to bake.

Analysis

Where a choice of ingredients is given in a recipe, the first one listed is the one we use in our analysis of nutritional value.

Breakfasts

For a good start to a great day, make sure you have breakfast. We've given ideas from leisurely Sunday breakfasts to simple quick ideas for the weekday rush. Breakfast can be as simple as a bowl of cereal and a serving of fruit, or as beguiling as a fruit platter followed by mouth-watering pancakes.

Start your day with plenty of carbohydrate and fiber. Begin with a breakfast cereal. This can be homemade or you can choose from the excellent commercial products available (see page 32). Hot cereal makes a terrific start to the day and lends itself to interesting toppings such as raisins, diced raw apple, cinnamon, or nuts.

Make your own breakfast blend using: oats, all-bran; wheat germ; bran (all sorts—rice, corn, oat, barley or wheat); dried fruits of every kind; unsalted raw nuts; seeds (pumpkin, sesame, linseed and sunflower); millet; buckwheat; puffed rice, wheat or corn; and wheatflakes. Serve with hot or cold skim or low-fat milk, yogurt and fruit.

With toast or bread, look at the toppings and fillings suggested on page 71. Consider the recipes for Date and Fig Spread, Strawberry Spread, and Dried Apricot Conserve in this section.

Fruit cleanses the palate and provides vitamins and minerals as well as carbohydrate and fiber. Eat it fresh, stewed or canned without added sugar. Combine fruits, top them with low-fat yogurt, cottage or ricotta cheese, or add them to cereal, or eat them on their own.

Cooked breakfasts are a pleasant treat. They need not take long to prepare. Try:

- Baked beans with freshly chopped mushrooms or green pepper
- Tomatoes, asparagus, mushrooms, or sweetcorn on toast
- Poached, scrambled, or boiled eggs
- Omelettes with fillings such as low-fat cheese and herbs, tomato combined with lean ham and onion, or a mushroom sauce

Meg's Muesli

Makes: approx 13.5 cups

4 cups rolled oats or barley
2 cups shredded coconut
1 cup raisins
1 cup unsalted cashews,
  chopped
2 cups unprocessed bran
2 cups All-Bran cereal
1½ cups wheatgerm

You can develop your own muesli recipe according to taste, but be very careful about the ingredients you add—check them against the nutritional listing on the packages to find out whether the additional ingredients you want to use have more fat than we recommend. Watch out, too, for added sugar.

1. Mix all ingredients well with a large spoon.

Nutritional data per ⅓ cup serving:
112 Calories, Carbohydrates 12g, Protein 4g, Fat 6g.

Exchanges per serving: 1 Starch, 1 Fat.

Preparation time: 15 minutes.

Dried Apricot Conserve

Makes: 1 cup

1 cup dried apricots
juice of 1 orange
pinch cinnamon
pinch ground cloves
½ cup warm water

You can vary this delectable yet simple recipe by using a dried fruit medley, dried peaches, or dried pears. You can also replace the cloves with fresh or ground ginger.

1. Chop apricots roughly.

2. Combine in mixing bowl with juice, spices, and water. Cover. Allow to stand 1 hour.

3. Spoon into saucepan and cook gently for approximately 10 minutes over low heat, stirring constantly, until mixture thickens and starts to combine. Alternatively, spoon into a bowl and microwave on high for 5 minutes. Stir two or three times during cooking until mixture thickens and starts to combine.

4. Spoon into container, cover and cool.

5. Stir again, adding a little more water if necessary, then refrigerate until ready to use.

To store: Cover and refrigerate for up to two weeks.

Nutritional data per 1 Tbsp. serving:
18 Calories, Carbohydrates 4g, Protein 0.5g, 0 Fat.

Exchanges per serving: ¼ Fruit.

Preparation time: 1½ hours.
Cooking equipment: small saucepan or microwave dish.

Breakfast in a Glass

Serves: 4

2 cups skim or low-fat milk
1 cup low-fat yogurt
3 ripe bananas or 1 cup
   fresh strawberries or
   unsweetened canned
   peaches or apricots
2 eggs (optional)
Equal or other artificial
   sweetener, to taste
Garnish:
ground allspice,
   cinnamon or nutmeg

If you simply don't have a moment in the morning, this quick breakfast comes in a glass.

1. Place all ingredients in a blender or food processor and blend well.

2. Serve at once, topped with a sprinkling of spice.

Nutritional data per serving:
179 Calories, Carbohydrates 26g, Protein 12g, Fat 4g.

Exchanges per serving: ³⁄₄ Milk, ³⁄₄ Fruit.

Preparation time: 5 minutes.
Equipment: food processor or blender.

Date and Fig Spread

Makes: 2 cups

1 cup seedless dates
1 cup dried figs
6 tsp lemon juice
¼ cup orange juice

The dates and figs have all the sweetness you need as a substitute for traditional sugar-laden jams.

1. Chop fruit finely.

2. Add to bowl, pour juice over, cover and soak overnight.

3. Spoon into blender or food processor and blend for approximately 2 minutes until smooth.

4. Store, covered, in a jar in refrigerator.

To store: Cover and refrigerate up to two weeks.

Nutritional data per 1 Tbsp. serving:
25 Calories, Carbohydrates 6g, Protein 0.3g, 0 Fat.

Exchanges per serving: ¹⁄₃ Fruit.

Preparation time: 15 minutes plus overnight soaking.
Cooking equipment: food processor or blender.

Fresh Strawberry Conserve

Makes: 1 cup

½ pint strawberries, hulled and roughly chopped
1 tbsp water
1 tbsp lemon juice
1 level tsp gelatin soaked in 1½ tbsp water
2 packets Equal or other artificial sweetener equivalent to 4 level tsp sugar

You can vary this recipe by using other berries instead of strawberries.

1. Place strawberries in saucepan with water and lemon juice.
2. Cover, bring to boil and simmer for 10 minutes, or microwave on high for 5 minutes.
3. Mash fruit slightly and let stand for 10 minutes.
4. Dissolve gelatin according to instructions on packet, and add to fruit.
5. Stir in sweetener.
6. Pour into a clean hot jar. Cover, cool and refrigerate.

To store: Cover and refrigerate for up to two weeks.

Nutritional data per 1 Tbsp. serving:
5 Calories, Carbohydrates 0.4g, Protein 0.2g, 0 Fat.

Exchanges per serving: Free food.

Preparation time: 30 minutes.
Cooking equipment: small saucepan.

Soft-Boiled Egg

Serves: 1

1 egg
1 slice whole wheat bread
½ tsp margarine
pepper
pinch salt

1. Bring water to boil in saucepan, lower egg in gently and soft boil to preference (3-5 minutes).
2. Crumble bread into an individual serving bowl.
3. Add margarine, pepper, and salt.
4. Lift egg out of water, crack open top, and spoon soft egg onto bread mixture.
5. Stir together gently and serve.

Variation: Add ½ tsp of finely chopped chives or parsley at step 3.

Nutritional data per serving:
145 Calories, Carbohydrates 10g, Protein 8g, Fat 8g.

Exchanges per serving: 1 Medium-Fat Meat, 1 Starch, ½ Fat.

Preparation time: 10 minutes.
Cooking equipment: small saucepan.

Appetizers and Snacks

Here we give you some ideas for quick and light meals, cocktail parties and pre-dinner hors d'oeuvres. Remember the basic principles of low fat when planning appetizers and snacks. The recipes in this section are also a useful source of carbohydrate which you can use to balance your daily meal plan.

If you are overweight, be careful not to over-indulge in these tempters.

Breads, like pumpernickel or rye, or whole wheat crackers make a good base for appetizers. Here are a few ideas:

Accompaniments for Dips

Vegetables: carrot sticks, cauliflower and broccoli florets, celery sticks, cucumber wedges, green or red bell pepper pieces, mushroom (button or slices), radish wedges, shallots.

Fruits: apple wedges tossed in lemon juice to prevent browning, cantaloupe or honey dew melon cut into chunks, kiwi wedges, fresh pineapple pieces, pear slices, fresh apricot halves.

Bread and biscuits: crusty whole wheat bread, dark rye or pumpernickel slices, triangles of toast, pita bread triangles (fresh or toasted), plain dry crackers, or crispbread.

Asparagus Rolls:

To serve four, you will need three slices of whole wheat bread and three slices of white high-fiber bread. Cut off the crusts and use a rolling pin to flatten the bread a little. Spread with margarine very lightly and place a spear of cooked fresh asparagus or canned asparagus diagonally across each slice of bread. Roll the bread towards a corner, press lightly to seal the edges of the bread. Cut each in half. Finally, garnish with rings of green or red bell pepper and parsley.

Pumpernickel Hors D'Oeuvres:

Many different combinations can be used to top rounds or squares of pumpernickel to make interesting and tasty hors d'oeuvres. Try these ideas:

- Baby prawns or shrimps and avocado
- Smoked salmon slices or rolls garnished with capers
- Sliced hard-boiled egg topped with black caviar and tiny sprigs of parsley
- Circles or squares of lean ham with asparagus tips
- Low-fat cottage cheese topped with strawberry halves or slices of peach or nectarine

Sandwich Fillings

Remember when you use any of these delicious fillings you do not need to use margarine on the bread—and use whole wheat bread rather than white. Use fillings for open sandwiches.

Cheese and . . .

- A mixture of grated low-fat Cheddar cheese, grated apple, carrot, chopped celery and pecans or walnuts; blend with Creamy Yogurt Dressing (page 188)

- Ricotta cheese with sliced cucumber, tomato, and chopped basil

- Ricotta cheese with chopped celery and walnuts

- Grated low-fat Cheddar cheese and sliced olives; blend with mustard

- Sliced low-fat Cheddar cheese, thinly sliced green apple, and Fresh Mango Chutney (page 189)

Egg and . . .

- Scrambled eggs with finely chopped lean ham

- Hard-boiled eggs mashed with alfalfa or bean sprouts and Curry Dressing (page 187)

Fish and . . .

- Salmon or tuna in water, with sliced cucumber or celery, topped with Creamy Yogurt Dressing (page 188)

- Shrimp, ricotta cheese, and thinly sliced cucumber

- Smoked salmon, low-fat cream cheese, and capers

Meat or Chicken and . . .

- Fresh Mango Chutney (page 189) or mustard topped with thinly sliced cold lean meat

- Chopped chicken, chives, and parsley blended with Creamy Yogurt Dressing (page 188)

- Chopped chicken, walnuts, and celery or green bell pepper, blended with low-fat natural yogurt

- Whole seed mustard, chopped lean ham, and grated apple

- Chopped chicken topped with thinly sliced raw mushrooms and Curry Dressing (page 187)

Vegetables and . . .

- Canned baked beans, lightly mashed and seasoned with Tabasco sauce

- Peanut butter and sliced cucumber or chopped celery

- Mashed kidney or three-bean mix with chili, bell pepper, cucumber, and onion

Sweet Fillings and . . .

- Mashed banana, lemon juice, and cinnamon

- Cottage or ricotta cheese with chopped dried figs

Chicken Liver Pâté

Serves: 6

8 oz chicken livers
¼ cup water
1 sprig fresh or ¼ tsp
  dried thyme
2 bay leaves
coarsely ground black
  pepper to taste
salt, to taste
½ cup port wine
Garnish:
coarsely ground black
  pepper

Chicken liver pâté is usually made with lots of butter and cream. This recipe avoids additional fats, yet tastes delicious.

1. Wash, dry and roughly chop the livers, discarding any greenish portions (these are not a sign of deterioration, but may discolor the pâté).

2. In saucepan, bring water to a boil. Add the liver and stir until sealed, about 2 minutes.

3. Add the thyme, bay leaves, pepper and salt. Cover, reduce heat and simmer gently for 10 minutes.

4. Add port wine and simmer, uncovered, a further 3 minutes.

5. If using fresh thyme, remove and discard the sprig. Remove and discard bay leaves.

6. Allow mixture to cool slightly. Purée liver and cooking liquids in a food processor or blender.

Variation: Replace port with 4 tbsp each of orange juice and brandy and add the grated rind of half an orange.

To store: Cover and refrigerate for up to three days.

To serve: As an appetizer: spoon the pâté into a serving bowl, sprinkle with black pepper, and chill for at least 1 hour before serving. Surround the dip with sliced fresh vegetables, crackers or triangles of dry toast.

As an entrée: Spoon the pâté into small, individual pots or ramekins. Smooth over the surface, sprinkle with black pepper and chill for at least 1 hour before serving. Place the pots on small plates and arrange a couple of dry toast triangles or crackers on each plate.

Nutritional data per serving (6 servings as appetizer):
98 Calories, Carbohydrates 3g, Protein 9g, Fat 3g.

Exchanges per serving: 1⅓ Lean Meat.

Preparation time: 30 minutes.
Cooking equipment: heavy-based saucepan, food processor or blender.

Moong Dhal

You can also serve this dip as a soup if you dilute it with 2 cups of chicken stock.

Makes: 2 cups

1 cup dried red lentils
3 cups water
½ tsp turmeric
1 tomato, peeled and chopped
2 tsp oil
½ tsp cumin seeds
3 curry leaves (optional)
1 onion, finely chopped or minced
2 cloves garlic, finely chopped or minced
1 tbsp ginger, chopped or finely minced
1½ tbsp Curry Powder (page 191), or to taste
½ cup boiling water (optional)
salt (optional)
Garnish:
1 tbsp chopped coriander (optional)

1. Wash lentils thoroughly, removing those that float.

2. Add 3 cups of water, turmeric, and chopped tomato, and boil mixture for 20-30 minutes until lentils are soft and the consistency is thick.

3. Heat oil in frying pan, add cumin seeds, curry leaves, onion, garlic, and ginger and sauté until golden. Stir in curry powder and sauté for 3-4 minutes more. If mixture is too thick, add about ½ cup of boiling water. Add this to the cooked lentils and stir well. Add salt if desired.

4. Just before serving, garnish with chopped coriander. Serve hot as a dip with accompaniments (see list, page 69).

Microwave method: Cook lentils on high for 20 minutes, otherwise follow the conventional recipe.

To store: Cover and refrigerate for up to two days. Reheat before serving.

Nutritional data per ¼ cup serving:
96 Calories, Carbohydrates 15g, Protein 7g, Fat 1.4g.
Exchanges per serving: 1 Starch, 1 Very Lean Meat.
Preparation time: 1 hour.
Cooking equipment: saucepan, frying pan.

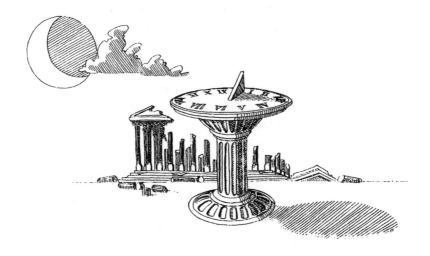

Dolmades

Serves: 4-6

2 cups Chicken Stock (see recipe on page 80)

1 cup basmati rice, uncooked

1 8-oz. chicken breast, skinned and ground or finely chopped

1 pkt preserved vine leaves

$\frac{1}{2}$ tsp cardamom, freshly crushed

$\frac{1}{2}$ tsp salt or 1 chicken stock cube

2 tsp olive oil and 2 tsp extra

1 lemon and juice of $\frac{1}{2}$ lemon extra

$\frac{1}{2}$ small finely chopped onion

Garnish:

2 tbsp chopped parsley

1. Bring chicken stock to a boil, reduce heat and simmer.
2. Wash rice and add to the stock.
3. Add chicken. Simmer gently, with lid on, until liquid is absorbed and rice is tender. Add more liquid (water) if necessary. Remove from heat.
4. Rinse vine leaves carefully to remove preserving liquid. Drain.
5. To rice mixture, add flavorings, 2 teaspoons oil, grated rind and juice of 1 lemon, onion, and parsley.
6. Place approximately 1 tablespoon of mixture on each vine leaf. Wrap firmly into parcels and place in a baking dish. Continue until all the vine leaves are used. Make sure dolmades are firmly packed into dish.
7. Pour a little water into the baking dish until it reaches about $\frac{1}{2}$ inch up the side of the dish. Squeeze juice of $\frac{1}{2}$ lemon over, and sprinkle extra 2 teaspoons olive oil over.
8. Cover with aluminium foil, and bake for about 1 hour.
9. Cool. Remove to a serving dish and serve garnished with parsley.

Accompaniment: Cucumber and Yogurt Sauce (page 184).

To store: Cover and refrigerate for up to three days. Do not store in an aluminum container.

Nutritional data per serving (if 4 servings):
151 Calories, Carbohydrates 15g, Protein 9g, Fat 6g.

Exchanges per serving: 1 Starch, $1\frac{1}{4}$ Very Lean Meat, 1 Fat.

Preparation time: 2 hours.
Cooking equipment: saucepan, baking dish.
Oven temperature: 325°F

Chick Pea Savory

Makes: 3 cups

1 cup of dried chick peas
water
2 tsp oil
2 large onions, chopped
2 tsp crushed garlic
2 tsp minced fresh ginger
1/2 tsp turmeric
1 tsp garam masala (see
  Indian Spices inset on
  page 157)
2 large ripe tomatoes,
  chopped
2 bay leaves
2 tbsp chopped fresh
  coriander or mint
lemon juice to taste
salt, to taste (optional)

Great served with chappati or flat bread.

1. Cover the chick peas with water and soak overnight.

2. In a saucepan, heat oil and sauté onion, garlic, and ginger until golden, stirring frequently. Add turmeric, garam masala, tomatoes, bay leaves, and half of fresh herbs. Add chick peas and soaking liquid, cover, and simmer on low heat until peas are tender. Set aside 1 tbsp of cooked chick peas for the garnish.

3. Remove bay leaves. Blend cooked chick peas in food processor or blender until smooth. Add lemon juice and salt if desired.

4. Sprinkle with remaining fresh herbs and the reserved tablespoon of unpuréed chick peas.

Nutritional data per 1/4 cup serving:
62 Calories, Carbohydrates 6g, Protein 2.4g, Fat 3.2g.

Exchanges per serving: 1/2 Starch, 1/2 Lean Meat.

Preparation time: 1 1/2 hours plus overnight.
Cooking equipment: saucepan, food processor, or blender.

Cheese Puffs

Serves: 4

2 eggs
2 thin slices lean ham,
  chopped
3 oz low-fat Cheddar
  cheese, grated
1 small firm tomato,
  finely chopped
1/2 tsp chopped chives
freshly ground black pepper
4 slices whole wheat
  bread

1. Preheat grill.
2. Place eggs in bowl and beat lightly with a fork.
3. Add remaining ingredients, except bread, and mix.
4. Toast bread on one side, remove from the grill and spread the cheese mixture over the untoasted side of the bread.
5. Grill until the mixture puffs up and browns. Serve hot.

Nutritional data per puff:
187 Calories, Carbohydrates 10g, Protein 14g, Fat 10g.

Exchanges per serving: 1 1/4 Lean Meats,
1/2 Medium-Fat Meat, 1/4 Vegetable, 1 Starch.

Preparation time: 15 minutes.

Vegetable Samosas

Serves: 4-8

1-2 per serve

2 medium potatoes,
  scrubbed and diced
1 medium carrot,
  scrubbed and diced
½ medium sweet
  potato, peeled and
  diced
1 cup frozen peas
1 medium onion, finely
  chopped
1 tsp olive oil
½ tsp turmeric
2 tsp Curry Powder
  (page 191)
½ tsp coriander
½ tsp salt or
  ½ Chicken Stock cube
1 tsp finely chopped or
  minced fresh ginger
pepper to taste
7 oz low-fat yogurt
12 sheets filo pastry
Garnish:
Sliced cucumber, onion and
  tomato

Count on serving one or two samosas per person.

1. Boil, steam, or microwave vegetables, except onion, until tender. Cool.

2. Sauté onion in oil until transparent but not brown. Combine with cooked vegetables in a bowl. Add spices. Check flavor and adjust to taste.

3. Using a pastry brush, spread a sheet of filo pastry lightly with yogurt. Place a second sheet over the first and repeat the procedure. Place a third sheet over this, then cut the pastry in half lengthwise with a sharp knife.

4. Place a generous spoonful of the vegetable mixture on one end of the pastry rectangle and fold the filo diagonally to cover the filling. Continue to fold diagonally until all the pastry is folded, making sure that the mixture is totally enclosed.

5. Repeat this procedure until all the pastry is used.

6. Place samosas on a baking sheet. Bake for approximately 15 minutes until brown. Serve with a garnish of sliced cucumber, onion and tomato.

Nutritional data per serving (if 4 servings):
252 Calories, Carbohydrates 44g, Protein 11g, Fat 4g.

Exchanges per serving: 2 Starch, 1½ Vegetable,
¼ Fat (mono), ¼ Milk.

Preparation time: 1 hour.
Cooking equipment: saucepan, frying pan, oven tray.
Oven temperature: 350°F.

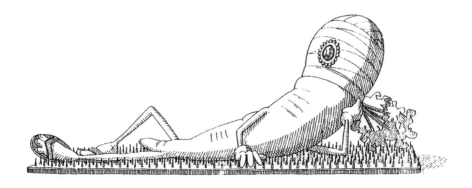

Whole Wheat Salmon Slices

Serves: 8

15 oz can pink salmon
4 oz ricotta cheese
juice of 1 lemon
1 tsp curry powder
¼ tsp salt
6 shallots, chopped
1 tsp gelatin
2 tbsp hot water
1 whole wheat baguette

Eat this on the day you make it because it does not keep. Use the soft bread from the center of the breadstick to make breadcrumbs.

1. Drain juice from salmon and discard skin and bones.
2. Mash the salmon and mix well with the cheese.
3. Add lemon juice, curry powder, salt, and shallots.
4. Melt gelatin in hot water, cool slightly, and stir into salmon mixture.
5. Chill in refrigerator for 30 minutes.
6. Cut baguette into two equal lengths, and remove the crusty ends. Hollow out with knife or spoon. Discard the soft centre.
7. Spoon filling into centres of breadstick and pack in firmly.
8. Wrap in aluminium foil and chill until ready to serve.
9. Slice in ¾ inch pieces and serve.

Nutritional data per serving:
143 Calories, Carbohydrates 6g, Protein 15g, Fat 7g.

Exchanges per serving: 2 Lean Meat, ½ Starch.

Preparation time: 45 minutes.

Mushroom Starter

Makes: 1 cup

¾ cup finely chopped
  mushrooms
1 tbsp chopped parsley
1 tsp finely chopped chives
¼ tsp ground oregano
  or ½ tsp of finely
  chopped fresh oregano
ground black pepper
¼ cup low-fat yogurt
salt, to taste

1. Mix all ingredients and refrigerate for 3 hours before serving.
2. Serve with cut-up fresh vegetables, breads, or crackers.

Nutritional data per ¼ cup serving:
17 Calories, Carbohydrates 1.7g, Protein 2.2g, Fat 0.25g.

Exchanges per serving: ½ Vegetable.

Preparation time: 10 minutes.

Chinese Dumplings

Makes: 4 servings

7 oz lean ground pork
4 shallots, finely chopped
8 oz can bamboo shoots, finely chopped
½ tsp minced ginger
1 tbsp low-sodium soy sauce
1 egg white
4 oz won ton pastry squares

Sauce for dipping
¼ cup soy sauce with dash of chili sauce

The won ton pastry squares used in this recipe are available from Asian food stores and some supermarkets.

1. Combine all ingredients except won ton pastry squares.
2. Place a heaping teaspoonful of mixture onto each won ton pastry square; keep unused pastry covered with a damp dish towel while you are working.
3. Squeeze the pastry up around the filling to make a filled-bag shape.
4. Place dumplings in an oiled steamer and cook over boiling water for approximately 20 minutes.
5. Serve with dipping sauce.

To store: Wrap well and freeze after they are cooked. Frozen dumplings can be thawed in the microwave. Place them in a covered microwave dish with 2 tbsp water.

Nutritional data per serving (4 dumplings per serving): 181 Calories, Carbohydrates 23g, Protein 17g, Fat 2g.

Exchanges per serving: 2 Lean Meat, 1 Vegetable, 1 Starch, ¼ Fat.

Preparation time: 45 minutes.
Cooking equipment: steamer, saucepan.

Chicken Spread

Makes: 1 cup

1 cup chopped cooked chicken
½ cup almonds or walnuts, chopped
juice of ½ lemon
3 tbsp low-fat yogurt
pinch mustard powder
1 tbsp chopped onion
1 tbsp chopped parsley

1. Blend all ingredients and refrigerate until ready to serve.
2. Serve on triangles of whole wheat toast, or roll in lettuce to make parcels.

To store: Cover and refrigerate up to two days.

Nutritional data per ¼ cup serving: 190 Calories, Carbohydrates 2g, Protein 17g, Fat 13g.

Exchanges per serving: 2 Lean Meat, 1 Fat.

Preparation time: 15 minutes.
Cooking equipment: blender or food processor.

Soups

Minestrone

2 medium onions
2 medium carrots
2 sticks celery
½ bell pepper
2 medium potatoes
4 oz green beans, sliced
1 cup shredded cabbage,
4 large tomatoes
2 tsp olive oil
1 cup dried cannellini
  beans
4 cups water
3 bay leaves
½ tsp salt
¼ tsp pepper
juice of ½ lemon
1 tsp dried mixed herbs
  or 2 tsp fresh mixed
  herbs

There are dozens of versions of this soup. This one has all the key ingredients of the classic version. To make this soup into a meal-in-one, you can add two cups of cooked pasta just before serving. This provides even more carbohydrate.

1. Peel and chop vegetables.

2. Heat oil in saucepan.

3. Add onions and cook until lightly browned.

4. Add carrots, celery, bell pepper, and potatoes. Cook until lightly colored.

5. Now add green beans, cabbage, and tomatoes. Cook until just tender.

6. Add dried beans, water, herbs, and lemon juice.

7. Simmer with lid on until beans are tender (approximately 1 hour).

8. Check for flavor and adjust to taste.

9. Serve with whole wheat breadsticks.

To store: Cover and refrigerate for up to three days.

Nutritional data per serving:
264 Calories, Carbohydrates 40g, Protein 17g, Fat 4g.

Exchanges per serving: 2 Vegetable, 2 Starch, ½ Fat, 1¼ Very Lean Meat.

Preparation time: 2 hours.
Cooking equipment: large saucepan or stock pot.

Chicken Stock

Makes: 4 cups

2 medium onions, peeled
1 large carrot
2 sticks celery
3 lb chicken parts
8 peppercorns
2 bay leaves
sprig of fresh or ¼ tsp
  dried thyme
5 sprigs parsley
6 cups water
salt, to taste

We've given storage options at the end of this recipe because chicken stock is so useful to have on hand. We use it in many other recipes, and it is superior to soup cubes or packet soups.

1. Wash and roughly chop the vegetables.
2. Place all the ingredients in a large saucepan.
3. Over medium heat, slowly bring mixture to a boil. Skim off any foam that rises to the surface. Reduce heat, cover saucepan, and simmer gently for 3 hours.
4. Strain the soup through a sieve. Reserve the meat for another dish. Discard skin, bones and vegetables.
5. Chill in refrigerator overnight and then skim off any congealed fat. Use in recipes requiring chicken stock or reheat and serve in cups as a nutritious hot beverage.

To store: Keep in a sealed container in refrigerator. Clarified stock will keep for three days if re-boiled every day. Freeze in an ice cube tray. Store cubes in a freezer bag for convenience.

Nutrition data per serving: negligible.

Preparation time: about 3 hours.
Cooking equipment: large saucepan.

Variation

Chicken Soup with Noodles or Rice

Just before serving, add half a cup of cooked vermicelli or boiled rice to the hot soup.

Green Pea, Spinach, and Chicken Soup

Serves: 4

2 cups frozen peas
3 cups Chicken Stock
(page 80)
8 oz pkt frozen spinach
1 cup chopped, cooked
chicken
2 tsp curry powder

1. Cook peas in stock until tender (approximately 15 minutes).
2. Combine in food processor until partly broken down and return to saucepan.
3. Add spinach and simmer until the spinach is thoroughly heated (approximately 10 minutes).
4. Add chicken and curry powder; bring to a boil and serve.

To store: Cover and refrigerate for up to two days.

Nutritional data per serving:
160 Calories, Carbohydrates 15g, Protein 19g, Fat 3g.

Exchanges per serving: ³⁄₄ Starch, 1¹⁄₂ Lean Meat,
¹⁄₂ Vegetable.

Preparation time: 45 minutes.
Cooking equipment: saucepan, food processor or blender.

Corn Chowder

Serves: 4

2 tsp margarine
1 large onion, peeled
and chopped
2 medium potatoes, peeled
1 Chicken Stock cube
(page 80)
pinch mixed dried herbs or
¹⁄₂ tsp fresh mixed herbs
pepper to taste
15 oz can corn kernels
¹⁄₂ cup water
1¹⁄₂ cups skim or
low-fat milk
4 tsp cornstarch

1. Melt margarine in saucepan. Add onion and cook over low heat until translucent.
2. Cut potatoes into ¹⁄₂ inch cubes and add to onion in saucepan.
3. Add stock cube and herbs, pepper, corn and its liquid, and the water.
4. Cover and simmer until potatoes are tender (approximately 15 minutes). Now add milk.
5. In a small bowl, blend cornstarch with a little water to a smooth paste. Add to the soup.
6. Bring to a boil, then simmer until slightly thickened, stirring from time to time.
7. Sprinkle with parsley and serve.

Nutritional data per serving:
246 Calories, Carbohydrates 44g, Protein 8g, Fat 4g.

Exchanges per serving: 2¹⁄₂ Starch, ¹⁄₃ Skim Milk,
¹⁄₂ Fat (poly).

Preparation time: 45 minutes.
Cooking equipment: large
saucepan.

Hungarian Soup

Serves: 4

3 cups Chicken Stock
  (page 80)
1 cup finely shredded
  red cabbage or ¾ cup
  canned red cabbage,
  drained
3 small onions, thinly
  sliced
1 clove garlic, crushed
2 large tomatoes, peeled
  and quartered
1 large apple, peeled
  and chopped
coarsely ground black
  pepper, to taste
¼ tsp ground all spice
Garnish: chives

This is a simple, filling, and aromatic soup with just a hint of sweetness, ideal for cold winter nights. Eaten with whole wheat bread, it makes a warming supper. For the stock, either use good quality cubes or make your own according to our recipe on page 80.

1. Place stock in a large saucepan and bring to a boil.

2. Add all other ingredients.

3. Cover and simmer for 30 minutes.

4. Serve, garnished with a sprinkling of chopped chives.

To store: Cover and refrigerate for up to three days.

Nutritional data per serving:
51 Calories, Carbohydrates 10g, Protein 2g, Fat trace.

Exchanges per serving: 1 Vegetable, ½ Fruit.

Preparation time: 45 minutes.
Cooking equipment: saucepan.

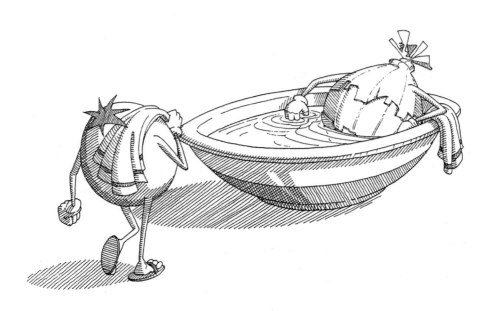

Hot and Sour Soup

Serves: 4

3 chicken breast fillets
   (1 lb)
2½ tbsp white vinegar
2 tsp oil
4 oz firm tofu cut into
   small cubes
4 cups Chicken Stock
   (page 80)
½ medium red bell
   pepper, cut into thin
   strips
4 oz button mushrooms
4 oz can bamboo shoots,
   drained
4 shallots, chopped
2 tbsp cornstarch
1 egg
Garnish: low-sodium soy
   sauce

1. With a sharp knife, slice chicken very finely.
2. Place chicken slices in bowl with vinegar.
3. Place oil in heavy saucepan and heat on high. Add tofu and stir-fry until tender (about 3 minutes). Remove from saucepan.
4. Pour chicken stock into saucepan with bell peppers, mushrooms, bamboo shoots, and shallots. Heat to boiling, cover and simmer 10 minutes or until vegetables are tender.
5. Add chicken and tofu, heat to boiling.
6. Mix cornstarch and a small amount of water in a separate bowl.
7. Slowly stir cornstarch mixture into boiling soup.
8. Cook, stirring constantly, until slightly thickened. Remove from heat.
9. Beat egg in a small bowl.
10. Then slowly pour egg mixture into soup, stirring quickly until egg swirls and has just set.
11. Spoon soup into individual bowls.
12. To each bowl add a dash of soy sauce.

To store: Cover and refrigerate for up to three days.

Nutritional data per serving:
317 Calories, Carbohydrates 8g, Protein 28g, Fat 19g.

Exchanges per serving: 4 Lean Meat, 1 Vegetable, 1 Fat.

Preparation time: 30 minutes.
Cooking equipment: large saucepan.

Singapore Noodle Soup

Serves: 4

10 oz green prawns
3 cups water
2 cups Chicken Stock
(page 80)
6 oz barbecued pork,
   lean
2 tsp sesame oil
2 cloves garlic, finely
   chopped
½ tsp ginger, finely
   chopped
3 oz fine egg noodles
1 cup bean sprouts,
   washed and drained
12 spinach leaves,
   washed and drained
½ tsp five spice powder
Garnish:
   3¼ oz can crab meat
   4 shallots, finely chopped
   ¼ cup finely diced
      cucumber

Although a soup, this dish makes an ideal light meal.

1. Shell and devein prawns. Wash shells and heads well and shake dry.

2. Bring water to boil, add shells and heads, cover and boil for 20 minutes. Strain.

3. Combine prawn stock and chicken stock.

4. Cut pork into thin strips.

5. Heat oil and gently fry garlic and ginger until starting to brown.

6. Add stock and prawns and simmer for 3 minutes.

7. Add noodles and simmer for a further 5 minutes.

8. Add pork, bean sprouts, spinach, and five spice powder and simmer for 2 minutes.

9. Pour into a large bowl and garnish with crab meat, shallots, and cucumber.

Nutritional data per serving:
334 Calories, Carbohydrates 19g, Protein 34g, Fat 13g.

Exchanges per serving: 4½ Lean Meat, ¾ Vegetable, ¾ Starch.

Preparation time: 45 minutes.
Cooking equipment: 1 large saucepan with lid.

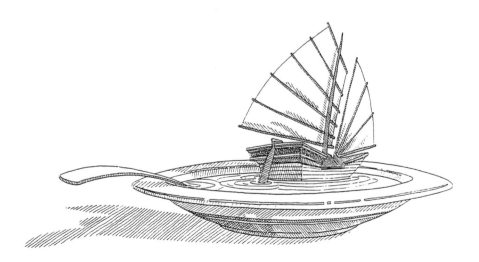

Chinese Chicken & Sweet Corn Soup

Serves: 4

2 tsp peanut oil
2 chicken breast fillets
 (10 oz), finely sliced
2 cloves garlic, crushed
1 tsp chopped ginger
1 quart Chicken Stock
 (page 80)
15 oz can creamed
 sweet corn
1 egg, lightly beaten
Garnish: 3 shallots,
 chopped

1. Place oil in saucepan and heat until moderately hot.

2. Lightly brown sliced chicken, garlic, and ginger. Don't overcook.

3. Add stock and bring to boil.

4. Add creamed corn and simmer for 10 minutes.

5. Remove from heat when ready to serve, then quickly stir in egg to make long strands.

6. Garnish with chopped shallots.

To store: Cover and refrigerate for up to three days.

Nutritional data per serving:
246 Calories, Carbohydrates 26g, Protein 17g, Fat 8g.

Exchanges per serving: $2^1/_2$ Lean Meat, $1^1/_2$ Starch.

Preparation time: 45 minutes.
Cooking equipment: saucepan.

Orange Borscht

Serves: 4

3 cups peeled and
 grated beets
3 cups Chicken Stock
 (page 80)
1 cup unsweetened
 orange juice
1 cup unsweetened
 tomato juice
1 sprig fresh thyme or
 $1/_4$ tsp dried thyme
ground black pepper
2 tbsp chopped parsley

Borscht is East European in origin and would, traditionally, have been eaten with plain boiled potatoes on the side. You can also add a spoonful of low-fat yogurt to each bowl just before you serve the soup.

1. Place beets and stock in saucepan and bring to a boil. Simmer for 20 minutes.

2. Strain stock into a clean saucepan and add 1 cup of the cooked beets. Discard the remaining beets.

3. Add the juices, thyme, and pepper.

4. Bring to boil and remove sprig of thyme.

5. Serve in bowls and sprinkle with chopped parsley.

To store: Cover and refrigerate for up to three days.

Nutritional data per serving:
63 Calories, Carbohydrates 13g, Protein 2g, Fat trace.

Exchanges per serving: 2 Vegetable, $1/_4$ Fruit.

Preparation time: 30 minutes.
Cooking equipment: 2 large saucepans.

Broccoli and Sweet Corn Soup

Serves: 4

1 large head broccoli
2 cups Chicken Stock
  (page 80)
15 oz can creamed
  sweet corn
1 stick celery, finely
chopped
6 shallots, finely sliced
½ tsp salt (optional)
pepper, to taste
Garnish: chopped chives

Note the high proportion of complex carbohydrate in this delicious soup.

1. Break the broccoli into florets and cook it in stock until tender (approximately 10 minutes).

2. Blend until smooth in food processor.

3. Add creamed sweet corn, celery, shallots, and seasonings.

4. Reheat and serve, garnished with chopped chives.

To store: Cover and refrigerate for up to three days.

Nutritional data per serving:
182 Calories, Carbohydrates 30g, Protein 9g, Fat 3g.

Exchanges per serving: 1¼ Starch, 2 Vegetable, ½ Fat.

Preparation time: 30 minutes.
Cooking equipment: saucepan, food processor or blender.

Curried Carrot and Rice Soup

Serves: 4

4 medium raw carrots,
  washed and chopped
1 onion, chopped
2 cups water
½ cup raw brown or
  basmati rice
1 cup water
2 tbsp finely chopped
  parsley
1 tsp curry powder
½ tsp salt
½ tsp black pepper
1½ cups skim milk
Garnish: paprika

Although we advocate as little salt as possible in our cooking, it seems to bring out the taste of all the other ingredients in curries.

1. Cook carrots and onions in 2 cups water until tender. Set aside in its cooking liquid.

2. In a second saucepan, cook rice in 1 cup water until tender (approximately 20–25 minutes). Drain and discard the cooking liquid.

3. Combine carrots, onions, and cooking liquid in food processor or blender until smooth. Add to parsley, curry powder, salt, pepper, cooked rice, and milk.

4. Return to saucepan and heat until just starting to boil.

5. Remove from the heat and serve, garnished with paprika.

Nutritional data per serving:
160 Calories, Carbohydrates 31g, Protein 7g, Fat 1g.

Exchanges per serving: 1 Starch, 1¼ Vegetable,
½ Skim Milk.

Preparation time: 1 hour.
Cooking equipment: 2 saucepans, food processor or blender.

Pork and Vegetable Noodle Soup

Serves: 4

7 oz soup bones
4 cups water
8 oz pork fillet, diced
1 medium carrot, grated
2 sticks celery, chopped
½ parsnip, grated
½ turnip, grated
1 medium leek, chopped
2 tbsp chopped parsley
½ tsp black pepper
3 oz pkt ramen noodles
Garnish: shallots, chopped

The noodles add complex carbohydrate to this nutritious soup.

1. Place soup bones and water in saucepan and bring to boil. Simmer for 1 hour. Strain stock and discard the bones.

2. Heat saucepan and fry pork fillet until browned.

3. Add pork, carrot, celery, parsnip, turnip, leek, parsley, and black pepper to stock.

4. Cook until meat and vegetables are tender.

5. Add noodles and cook a further 5-10 minutes or until noodles are tender, too.

6. Spoon into individual bowls, garnish with chopped shallots.

Nutritional data per serving:
151 Calories, Carbohydrates 16g, Protein 18g, Fat 2g.

Exchanges per serving: 2 Lean Meat, ¾ Vegetable, ¾ Starch.

Preparation time: 2 hours.
Cooking equipment: 2 saucepans.

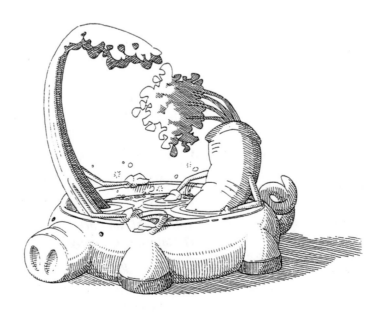

Souper Douper Pumpkin Soup

Serves: 4

1½ lb pumpkin, peeled,
  cut into pieces
1 large leek, sliced
3 cups Chicken Stock
  (page 80)
2 tsp mixed dried herbs
  or 3 tsp fresh herbs
½ tsp coarsely ground
  black pepper
¼ tsp ground nutmeg
¼ tsp coriander
½ tsp salt
2 tbsp lemon juice
2 tbsp chopped parsley

1. Place all ingredients except lemon juice and parsley in a saucepan.

2. Bring to a boil and simmer until pumpkin is tender (approximately 20 minutes).

3. Cool slightly, blend in food processor or blender until smooth.

4. Add lemon juice and parsley. Check taste, add salt if needed.

5. Serve with Herby Corn Muffins (page 219).

To store: Cover and refrigerate for up to three days.

Nutritional data per serving:
82 Calories, Carbohydrates 14g, Protein 5g, Fat 1g.

Exchanges per serving: ³⁄₄ Fruit, ¹⁄₄ Vegetable.

Preparation time: 1 hour.
Cooking equipment: saucepan, food processor or blender.

Gazpacho

Serves: 4

1 small cucumber, peeled
3 shallots
½ red and ½ green
  bell pepper
2 sticks of celery
4 med. ripe tomatoes or a
  15 oz can of tomatoes
1 medium white onion
1 cup tomato juice
1 tbsp coarsely ground
  black pepper
1-2 tsp Tabasco sauce,
Garnish: chopped parsley

1. Finely chop half the cucumber, 3 shallots, a quarter of each red and green bell pepper, a stick of celery and 1 tomato. Set aside.

2. Roughly chop all remaining vegetables and place in food processor with tomato juice, pepper, and Tabasco sauce and blend until smooth.

3. Add finely chopped vegetables, mix and chill well.

4. Serve, garnished with chopped parsley.

To store: Cover and refrigerate for up to three days.

Nutritional data per serving:
47 Calories, Carbohydrates 8g, Protein 3g, Fat trace.

Exchanges per serving: 2 Vegetable.

Preparation time: 25 minutes.
Cooking equipment: food processor or blender.

Beef and Bean Soup

Serves: 4

8 oz lean ground beef
1 medium onion, diced
1 small clove garlic
2 sticks celery, diced
14 oz can tomatoes
1 tbsp tomato paste
3 cups water
½ tsp oregano, dried, or
  1 tsp fresh
½ tsp paprika
½ tsp ground cumin
2 tsp white vinegar
15 oz can kidney beans,
  drained

This hearty soup only needs plenty of whole wheat bread to make it into a meal-in-one.

1. Fry meat, add onion and garlic and cook until juices evaporate and ground beef is well browned.

2. Add celery, tomatoes, tomato paste, water, oregano, paprika, cumin, and vinegar.

3. Bring to a boil. Add beans and reduce heat to low, cover and simmer 30 minutes.

To store: Cover and refrigerate for up to three days.

Nutritional data per serving:
202 Calories, Carbohydrates 17g, Protein 26g, Fat 3g.

Exchanges per serving: 3 Lean Meat, 1¼ Vegetable, ¾ Starch.

Preparation time: 1 hour.
Cooking equipment: saucepan.

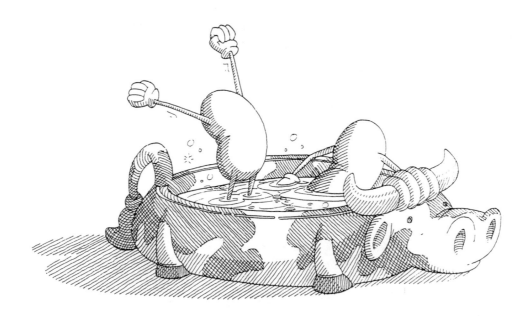

Entrées and Light Meals

Harlequin Noodle Salad

Serves: 4

1 cup shell pasta,
  uncooked
1 cup cooked and diced
  chicken
1/2 cup diced celery
1 small green and
  1 small red bell pepper,
  chopped
4 shallots, chopped
1 tbsp chopped parsley
1/2 cup raisins
black pepper, to taste
dressing: 1/2 quantity
  Curry Dressing (page 187)
Garnish: 4 lettuce cups

Make this the day before you want to serve it, so the flavor can develop.

1. Place pasta in saucepan of boiling water. Cook until tender and then drain.

2. Combine cooked pasta, diced chicken, celery, bell pepper, shallots, parsley, raisins, and black pepper.

3. Mix in the curry dressing.

4. Refrigerate for 1 hour.

5. Serve in lettuce cups.

To store: Keep in airtight container in refrigerator for up to two days.

Nutritional data per serving:
227 Calories, Carbohydrates 34g, Protein 16g, Fat 3g.
Exchanges per serving: 2 Very Lean Meat, 1 Fruit,
1/2 Vegetable, 1 Starch.

Preparation time: 1 1/2 hours plus preparation time
for dressing.
Cooking equipment: saucepan.

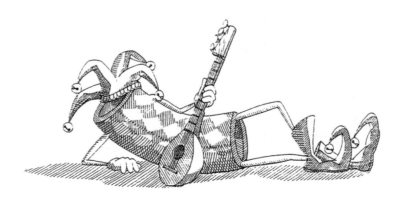

Whole Wheat Beef & Bean Burritos

Serves: 4

Filling:
1 lb lean ground beef
1 medium onion, chopped
1 beef stock cube or ½ tsp salt
½ tsp pepper
5 oz tomato paste
3 fl oz water
Tabasco sauce to taste
juice of ½ lemon
15 oz can red kidney beans, rinsed and drained

Tortillas:
1 cup each, whole wheat flour and unbleached flour
2 tsp baking powder
½ tsp salt
1 cup warm water
Garnish: shredded lettuce and finely chopped onion

Filling:

1. Fry meat until lightly browned. Add onion and continue to sauté until browned.

2. Add crumbled stock cube, pepper, tomato paste, water, Tabasco sauce, and lemon juice. Stir until well combined. Add kidney beans and mix in well. Bring to a boil, turn down the heat and simmer 10-15 minutes until the meat is cooked.

3. Add extra water, if necessary, to make a thick sauce.

4. Keep meat and bean mixture warm until tortillas are ready or allow to cool, refrigerate and reheat when needed.

Tortillas:

5. Sift flours, baking powder and salt.

6. Gradually stir in warm water to form a dough.

7. Turn dough onto floured board and knead until smooth. Cover with plastic film and allow to rest 15-20 minutes.

8. Cut into 12 equal pieces. Shape each into a ball.

9. Flatten each ball into a 4-5 inch patty, roll into a very thin, round pastry, approximately 9-10 inches, making sure dough and rolling pin are well floured to prevent sticking.

10. Heat frying pan. Place each tortilla on dry surface of frying pan. As blisters appear, press gently with spatula. When underside is brown, turn over and cook until blisters have formed on other side and tortilla is lightly browned.

11. Lift onto tray covered with a damp dish towel. Fold dish towel to cover tortilla.

12. Repeat until all tortillas are cooked.

13. Place some hot filling onto the center of each tortilla, and sprinkle lightly with lettuce and onion if desired. Roll up filled tortilla and serve immediately.

Nutritional data per serving:
533 Calories, Carbohydrates 66g, Protein 59g, Fat 7g.

Exchanges per serving: 3 Starch, 4 Lean Meat, 2 Vegetable.

Preparation time: 2 hours.
Cooking equipment: frying pan.

Prosciutto and Melon

Serves: 4

1 ripe cantaloupe, peeled
  and seeded
12 slices paper-thin lean
  prosciutto (3 ounces)
4 lettuce leaves

1. Cut melon into two and then each half into six pieces, evenly shaped to give 12 pieces.

2. Wrap each piece in a slice of prosciutto and secure with a toothpick.

3. Arrange lettuce leaves on four individual plates and top each with three pieces of melon and prosciutto. Serve chilled.

Nutritional data per serving:
45 Calories, Carbohydrates 4g, Protein 2g, Fat 2g.

Exchanges per serving: $^1/_4$ Fruit, $^1/_4$ Medium-Fat Meat.

Preparation time: 15 minutes.

Variation: use honey dew melon instead of cantaloupe if you wish. Try using smoked pork or smoked beef instead of prosciutto.

Spinach Ravioli
with Fresh Tomato Sauce

Serves: 4

6 large ripe tomatoes,
  roughly chopped
1 tsp sugar
1 tsp chopped fresh
  basil or $^1/_2$ tsp dried
  basil
pinch tarragon
12 oz fresh spinach
  ravioli
2 oz low-fat Cheddar
  cheese, grated

1. Place tomatoes, sugar, and herbs in saucepan and simmer gently until mixture forms a thick sauce.

2. While tomatoes are cooking, fill a second saucepan three-quarters full with cold water and rapidly bring to boil. Add ravioli and cook until tender. Drain.

3. Pour sauce over ravioli and mix gently.

4. Sprinkle with cheese.

Nutritional data per serving:
312 Calories, Carbohydrates 51g, Protein 15g, Fat 5g.

Exchanges per serving: $1^1/_2$ Vegetable, 1 Lean Meat, 3 Starch.

Preparation time: 45 minutes.
Cooking equipment: 2 saucepans.

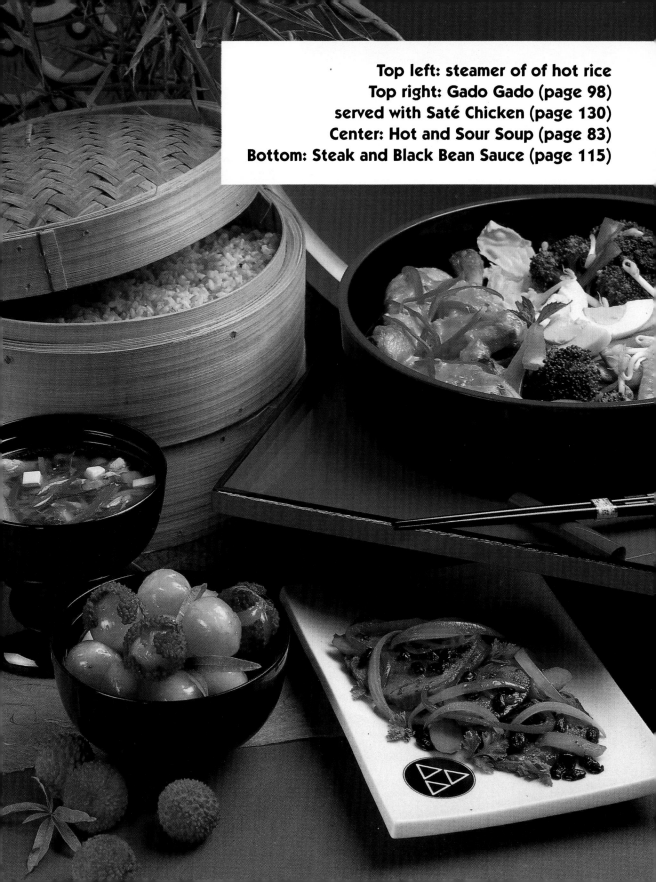

Top left: steamer of of hot rice
Top right: Gado Gado (page 98)
served with Saté Chicken (page 130)
Center: Hot and Sour Soup (page 83)
Bottom: Steak and Black Bean Sauce (page 115)

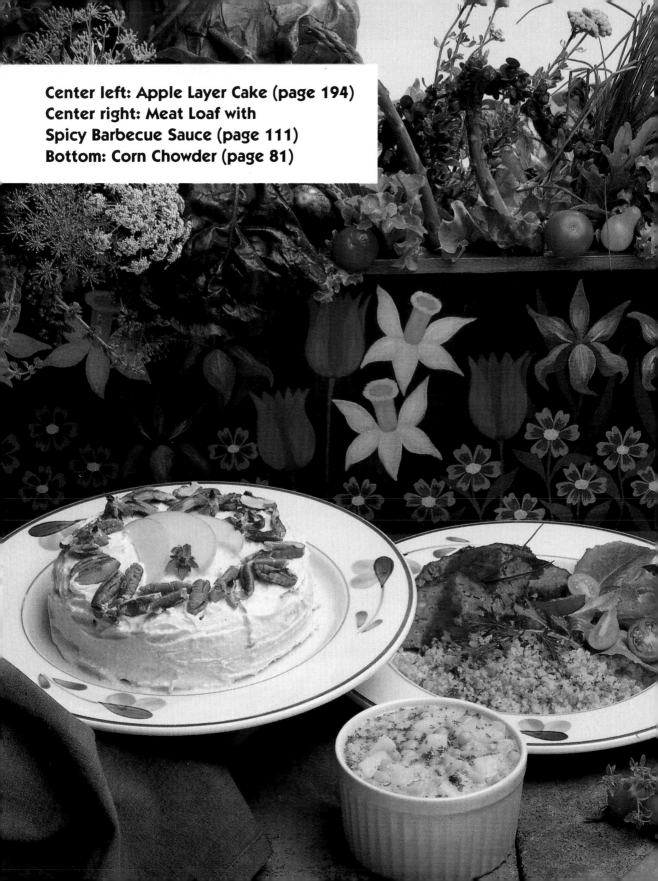

Center left: Apple Layer Cake (page 194)
Center right: Meat Loaf with
Spicy Barbecue Sauce (page 111)
Bottom: Corn Chowder (page 81)

Bombay Burgers
with Cucumber and Yogurt Sauce

Makes 12 patties

1 cup dried red lentils
1 large potato, cut into
  pieces
1 medium onion, finely
  chopped
¼ cup shredded coconut
1 tbsp sesame seeds
1 tbsp plain flour
1 tsp curry powder
1 tsp finely chopped
  fresh ginger
½ tsp salt
¼ tsp pepper
2 tsp lemon juice
¾–1 cup wheat germ or
  whole grain bread crumbs

Garnish:

sliced onion rings
1 cup Cucumber and
  Yogurt Sauce (page 184)

1. Soak lentils in water for 2 hours.

2. Rinse, cover with water in a saucepan and simmer for approximately 30 minutes until tender. Add potato 10 minutes into the cooking time. Alternatively, place lentils in a bowl with water and microwave on high for 20 minutes or until tender. Add potato 10 minutes into the cooking time.

3. Drain any liquid from lentils and potato, and mash thoroughly. Add onion, coconut, sesame seeds, flour, spices, and lemon juice.

4. Allow to cool (preferably chill).

5. Shape into patties and coat with wheatgerm or breadcrumbs.

6. Bake on lightly oiled tray for 10-15 minutes, or cook in a frying pan lightly brushed with oil, taking care not to burn the coating.

7. Serve hot garnished with onion rings and with Cucumber and Yogurt Sauce.

Nutritional data per serving:
200 Calories, Carbohydrates 22g, Protein 10g, Fat 8g.

Exchanges per serving: 1½ Starch, 1 Fat,
1 Very Lean Meat, ¼ Vegetable.

Preparation time: 1 hour plus preparation time for sauce.
Cooking equipment: saucepan, oven tray or frying pan.
Oven temperature: 375°F.

Crêpes

Serves: 4
Makes: 12 large or 24
small crêpes

1 cup whole wheat or
   unbleached flour or
   half and half
3 eggs, lightly beaten
2 tsp oil or melted butter
1½ cups skim milk

Crêpes are small, very thin pancakes; the raw batter is thinner than for traditional pancakes.

Pancakes make a large, hearty wrapping for a variety of fillings. The cooked pancake should be about ⅛ inch thick.

Both crêpes and pancakes are simple to make and very versatile. With either savory or sweet fillings, use them for entrées, main courses, desserts or snacks.

You will find that crêpes made entirely with whole wheat flour tend to be heavy. A half-and-half combination makes a nutritious and tasty version.

1. Using a food processor or blender, add all ingredients at once and process until smooth.

Working by hand, sift flour into a bowl (if using whole wheat flour, add any wheat husks left in sieve to the sifted flour). Make a well in the flour. Slowly add the beaten eggs, stirring continually to draw the ingredients together and prevent lumps forming. Mix oil or melted butter with milk. Slowly add to flour mixture, stirring continually, to form a thin, smooth pouring consistency like that of thin pouring cream. If too thick, add more milk, a little at a time, until you have the right consistency.

2. Transfer batter to a jug and leave to stand in a cool place for at least an hour. If the mixture has thickened, add more milk, a little at a time, to the consistency of thin pouring cream.

3. Lightly grease a crêpe or heavy-bottomed frying pan and heat until very hot, but not smoking. Pour in 2-4 tbsp of batter, depending on size of pan, tilt pan to spread batter evenly.

4. When fine bubbles appear on the surface of the crêpe and it appears dry, use a spatula to flip over and cook the other side for approximately 5 seconds until pale golden brown.

5. Repeat these steps for the remainder of the batter, brushing the pan with a little oil between crêpes and stacking them as they are cooked. Keep them covered with a damp dish towel until you need them.

Use any of the filling mixtures on page 96, or create your own. Crêpes can be filled and then served rolled up or folded in half or in quarters.

To store: Cover and refrigerate for up to two days, or pack in freezer bags, with a layer of waxed paper or plastic film between each crêpe, and freeze.

Nutritional data per serving (3 crêpes):
231 Calories, Carbohydrates 29, Protein 12g, Fat 7g.

Exchanges per serving: 1¼ Starch, ¾ Medium-Fat Meat, ½ Fat, ½ Milk.

Preparation time: batter 10 minutes, standing time for raw batter 1 hour, cooking time 20 minutes.
Cooking equipment: jug, crêpe pan or small frying pan.

Pancakes

Serves: 4-5
(makes 8-10 pancakes)

¾ cup whole wheat or
  unbleached flour or
  half-and-half
1 egg
1¼–1½ cups skim milk

This is a traditional recipe. Pancakes are larger and heavier-textured than crêpes. The pancakes should be about the size of a dinner plate and about ⅛ inch thick. The same guidelines we set out at the start of the crêpe recipe apply here.

1. Follow instructions as in previous crêpe recipe.

To store: As for crêpes.

Nutritional data per serving (2 pancakes):
103 Calories, Carbohydrates 20g, Protein 6g, Fat 0.5g.

Exchanges per serving: 1 Starch, ¼ Medium-Fat Meat, ¼ Milk.

Preparation time: batter 10 minutes, standing time for raw batter 1 hour, cooking time 20 minutes.
Cooking equipment: jug, small frying pan.

Savory Fillings
for Crêpes or Pancakes

Allow three crêpes or two pancakes per serving. Fill pancakes with any of the fillings that follow, and top with low-fat natural yogurt or ricotta cheese or a fine sprinkling of Parmesan cheese.

Serve the filled pancakes hot, accompanied by a crisp, green salad.

Ham and asparagus

Diced lean ham and cooked asparagus spears or pieces tossed in Cheese Sauce (page 181).

Mushroom and onion

Sliced mushrooms and onions cooked in a frying pan brushed with oil and tossed in White Sauce (page 178).

Ratatouille

Ratatouille Sauce (page 183) topped with grated low-fat Cheddar cheese.

Spinach

Cooked, chopped spinach mixed with ricotta cheese, sautéed shallots, chopped basil and pine nuts.

Seafood

1 lb seafood cooked in one quantity of Tomato and Basil Sauce (page 180).

Chicken and avocado

Two sliced, cooked, chicken fillets and one sliced avocado tossed in one quantity Cheese Sauce (page 181).

Savory beef

1 lb lean ground beef cooked in one quantity of Tomato and Basil Sauce (page 180).

Steak and onion

Slice 1 lb fillet steak into very thin strips, and marinate in 2 tbsp Worcestershire sauce and 1 crushed clove of garlic for 10 minutes. Sauté beef in 2 tsp oil for 3 minutes. Add 1 large sliced onion and sauté for another 2 minutes. Add ¼ cup red wine, and simmer for 1-2 minutes. Thicken with 1 tbsp cornstarch blended with 2 tbsp water. Fill pancakes and serve them topped with low-fat natural yogurt and a sprinkling of chopped parsley.

Red kidney bean and corn

Sauté 1 medium finely diced bell pepper and 1 medium finely chopped onion in 3 tbsp water for approximately 3 minutes until soft. Add 1 cup drained canned red kidney beans, 1 cup drained canned corn kernels, 2 tbsp tomato paste, ¼ tsp ground oregano and a small pinch chili powder. Simmer gently for 5-10 minutes until the liquid is almost evaporated. Fill the pancakes and roll them up. Sprinkle with 4 tbsp low-fat grated cheese, and grill to melt the cheese topping.

Pasties

7 oz rump, porterhouse,
or fillet steak
1 potato, finely diced
1 medium carrot, finely
diced
1 small turnip, finely diced
1 small onion, finely diced
$\frac{1}{4}$ tsp white pepper
$\frac{1}{4}$ tsp dried mixed herbs
2 tbsp finely chopped
parsley
1 quantity Whole Wheat
Pastry (page 218)
1 tbsp water
Glaze:
2 tbsp skim milk

Preparation time: 1$\frac{1}{2}$ hours.
*Cooking equipment: baking
tray.*
Oven temperature: 400°F.

*As a main course, serve pasties with vegetables and Tomato
and Basil Sauce (page 180). They also make a wonderful light
lunch or meal, served with salad.*

1. Cut meat into small cubes, about $\frac{1}{2}$ inch x $\frac{1}{2}$ inch.

2. In a bowl, combine meat, diced vegetables, pepper and
   herbs.

3. Divide pastry into four portions. Roll out each portion to
   about the size of a saucer.

4. Divide the meat mixture between the rounds, placing
   meat slightly off the center of each round.

5. Brush the edges of the pastry with a little water. Fold
   pastry over, in half, to make a half-moon shape.

6. Use back of fork to crimp the edges of the pasties firmly.

7. Place the finished pasties on a lightly greased baking tray.
   Prick the top of each pasty three times with a fork. Brush
   the surface of each pasty with a little skim milk.

8. Bake for 35 minutes or until browned.

To freeze: Prepare pasties to Step 6, place in freezer bags.
Defrost before baking, as above.

Nutritional data per serving:
567 Calories, Carbohydrates 56g, Protein 22g, Fat 28g.
Exchanges per serving: 1$\frac{3}{4}$ Medium-Fat Meats, 3 Starch,
1 Vegetable.

Variation:
Filo Rolls

*This variation of pasties keeps the fat content down—12 sheets
of filo pastry are all you need to make four rolls.*

1. Precook the meat and vegetables by combining them in
   a saucepan with $\frac{1}{2}$ cup of water and simmering them for
   10 minutes. Drain.

2. Use 3 sheets of filo pastry per roll, folding each sheet in
   half to make 6 layers. Brush skim milk between the layers
   of the filo pastry. Divide the meat mixture into 4 and
   place a portion on each portion of filo and roll them into

parcels. Brush the inner edges of the filo with a little skim milk and press down gently to seal. Glaze the tops of the rolls lightly with skim milk. Bake for 15-20 minutes, or until crisp and lightly brown.

To store: Cover and refrigerate for up to two days. Reheat slowly but thoroughly. If you want to freeze them, do so before you bake them. Later thaw and bake them as above.

Nutritional data per serving:
205 Calories, Carbohydrates 28g, Protein 16g, Fat 3g.

Exchanges per serving: 1³/₄ Medium-Fat Meats, 1¹/₂ Starch, 1 Vegetable.

Gado Gado

Serves: 4

1 cup bean sprouts
1 cup green beans
1¹/₂ cups broccoli florets
1 cup sliced carrots
1 cup diced cabbage
1 medium green
  bell pepper,
  sliced
6–10 snow peas
2 tomatoes, cut into
  wedges
2 onions, cut into wedges
1 small cucumber,
  peeled and diced
2 hard-boiled eggs, cut
  into quarters

You have free reign with this recipe to add or change vegetables according to season or taste.

1. Half fill a medium saucepan with water and bring to a rapid boil. Plunge the vegetables, except the tomatoes and cucumber, one variety at a time, into the boiling water for no more than 1 minute, or until the color intensifies, or microwave with 2 tbsp water on high for 2 minutes. Quickly remove the blanched vegetables from the water, place in a colander and immediately rinse with cold, running water; this preserves the color and crispness. Bring water back to a boil before blanching each type of vegetable.

2. Arrange all the ingredients on a platter.

3. Serve as an appetizer or entrée at either room temperature or chilled with cooked brown rice and a dish of warm Saté (Peanut) Sauce (page 179).

To store: Cover and refrigerate for no more than one day.

Nutritional data per serving:
103 Calories, Carbohydrates 10g, Protein 9g, Fat 3g.

Exchanges per serving: 2¹/₂ Vegetable,
¹/₂ Medium-Fat Meat.

Preparation time: 30 minutes.
Cooking equipment: medium saucepan, large saucepan.

Fish and Seafood

The beauty of fish and seafood is that they have plenty of protein, vitamins, and minerals and little fat. This makes them lower in calories than an equivalent serving of meat and makes fish and seafood an invaluable, and delicious, part of your regular meal plan.

COOKING FISH AND SEAFOOD

Baking

Whole fish (large or small), cutlets, or fish fillets are all equally good cooked this way. Place the fish in a shallow casserole and flavor it to taste, for instance with a sliced onion, a bay leaf, herbs of your choice and a few peppercorns, a little salt (optional). Then pour over the fish approximately ½–1 cup of liquid depending on the amount of fish. The liquid can be low-fat milk, wine, or tomato juice. Bake, covered, at 350°F for 15–20 minutes or until the fish flakes when you test it with a fork.

Alternatively, place the fish on foil, sprinkle with lemon juice and herbs, seal, and then cook as above without any additional liquid.

Grilling

Allow 5-8 minutes for fillets, cutlets, kebabs, or small fish; 10 minutes for medium-sized whole fish and 15-20 minutes for large whole fish. Watch the fish carefully while it grills, turning it once or twice, or it will overcook and dry out.

We have given some lovely marinade recipes in this book which you can use to flavor the fish before and use as a baste while cooking. Grilled fish is delicious cooked with no more than a sprinkling of herbs, lemon juice, black pepper, and a little salt (optional).

Poaching

With this method the fish cooks in a flavored, simmering liquid. Place the fish in a shallow saucepan with a lid, add just enough liquid (milk, stock, or wine, or a combination of any two of these) to barely cover the fish and then season it to taste. You can, for instance, add sliced onion, bay leaf, peppercorns, ground black pepper, parsley and a sliced carrot, which will give you a wonderfully flavorsome result. Add salt if you like.

Cover and simmer gently on the stove for 5–8 minutes if you are using thin fillets, or for about 10 minutes if you are using thicker pieces. Again, use the test of flaking the fish with a fork to check when it's ready and take it off the heat immediately. Use the poaching liquid as the base for sauce.

Microwaving

Fish and seafood are excellent cooked in the microwave. Place fish in the microwave dish, add ¼ cup of liquid such as wine, stock or low-fat milk, flavor as for poaching or baking above, cover with plastic wrap and cook the fish on high. Allow 3 minutes for small fillets, 5–7 minutes for larger fillets or small whole fish and 10–12 minutes for large whole fish. Arrange the seafood in a single layer in a shallow dish. Cover with plastic wrap and cook on medium until opaque (approximately 3–4 minutes). Let stand, covered, for 5 minutes before serving.

Fish with Various Sauces

Grill 4 fillets of white fish such as snapper, flathead, whiting, or sea perch on both sides until cooked through (approximately 8–10 minutes). Alternatively, cover and microwave on medium-high for 4–6 minutes. Serve topped with a sauce such as:

- Green Champagne (page 180)
- Ratatouille (page 183)
- Black Bean (page 183)
- Sweet and Sour (page 185)

Seafood Pasta

Serves: 4

10 oz pasta (spaghetti,
  tagliatelle, or macaroni)
2 tbsp water
½ med. onion, chopped
1 clove garlic, crushed
1 cup skim milk
2 tsp cornstarch
1½ cups mixed cooked
  seafood (oysters,
  calamari, shrimps,
  clams, scallops)
1 tbsp parsley, chopped
coarsely ground black
  pepper, to taste
salt, to taste

1. Fill a large saucepan two-thirds with water, and bring to a rapid boil. Add pasta, and boil rapidly for 10-12 minutes until *al dente* (tender, but still firm to bite).

2. While the pasta is cooking, prepare the sauce. In a medium saucepan, boil the 2 tablespoons of water. Add the onion and garlic and cook until tender.

3. In a small bowl, blend 1 tablespoon of the milk with the cornstarch to make a smooth paste. Then stir in the remainder of the milk. Add mixture to the onion and garlic, and stir constantly over medium heat until sauce thickens.

4. Over medium heat, add all the remaining ingredients, and stir to combine and heat through.

5. Drain the pasta and add to the sauce. Toss gently to combine.

6. Serve at once.

Nutritional data per serving:
357 Calories, Carbohydrates 48g, Protein 31g, Fat 4g.

Exchanges per serving: 3 Very Lean Meat, 3 Starch,
¼ Milk.

Preparation time: 30 minutes.
Cooking equipment: large saucepan, medium saucepan.

Fish in Orange Sauce

Serves: 4

juice of 2 oranges
juice of 1 lemon
1 tsp margarine
¼ tsp coarsely ground
  black pepper
4 fish fillets (6 oz each)
small quantity of flour

1. Place juices, margarine, and pepper in pan.

2. Cook until slightly reduced.

3. Dust fish with flour.

4. Add to sauce and poach until just cooked, turning once.

5. Lift out onto serving plates. Spoon sauce over.

Nutritional data per serving:
166 Calories, Carbohydrates 4g, Protein 27g, Fat 4g.

Exchanges per serving: 4 Very Lean Meat, ¼ Fruit.

Preparation time: 15 minutes.
Cooking equipment: frying pan.

Curried Tuna and Rice Casserole

Serves: 4

15 oz tuna canned
  in water
juice of 1 lemon
4 oz raw brown rice
Sauce:
2 small onions, diced
3 tsp curry powder
2 tbsp whole wheat flour
3 cups skim milk
2 slices whole wheat
  bread, crumbed

Replace tuna with salmon if you prefer.

1. Mix tuna and lemon juice in bowl.
2. Cook brown rice in boiling water according to package directions.
3. Drain rice and combine with the tuna mixture.
4. Fry onion and curry powder in a saucepan.
5. Combine flour with enough milk to make a smooth paste.
6. Add remaining milk to onions and curry powder and bring to a boil. Remove from heat and add the flour paste.
7. Return to heat and stir continually until mixture thickens.
8. Pour two-thirds of the curry sauce over tuna and rice. Mix.
9. Spoon into a casserole, pour remaining sauce over the top.
10. Cover with breadcrumbs, and bake in the oven until golden and the casserole is heated through (approx. 30 minutes).

To store: Cover and refrigerate for 24 hours.

Nutritional data per serving:
365 Calories, Carbohydrates 45g, Protein 36g, Fat 4g.

Exchanges per serving: 4 Very Lean Meat, 2½ Starch, ¾ Skim Milk.

Preparation time: 1 hour 40 minutes.
Cooking equipment: 2 saucepans, casserole.
Oven temperature: 325°F.

Piquant Fish in Foil

Serves: 4

4 large fish fillets (6 oz
  each), or small whole fish
2 tsp finely chopped,
  fresh tarragon or
  ½ tsp dried
1 tbsp very finely
  chopped parsley
  (optional)
coarsely ground black
  pepper, to taste
1 medium onion, thinly
  sliced
1 lemon, thinly sliced
juice of 1 lemon
2 tbsp dry white wine
  (optional)

This is a wonderful way to prepare fresh fish. Serve it with baked potatoes and a crisp salad.

1. Use four pieces of foil large enough to completely wrap the fish fillets. Lightly grease the foil or spray it well with non-stick cooking spray.
2. Place the fish fillets on the pieces of foil. Sprinkle each fillet with the herbs and black pepper. Arrange several onion rings on top of each fillet and top with one or two slices of lemon.
3. Mix lemon juice and white wine and pour over the fish.
4. Wrap each fillet in foil, sealing along the top, so that the juices aren't lost during cooking or when opening the foil.
5. Place the foil parcels, sealed side up, on a baking tray. Bake or barbecue for 30 minutes.
6. Open foil along the sealing edge and serve immediately.

Nutritional data per serving:
149 Calories, Carbohydrates 2g, Protein 27g, Fat 3g.

Exchanges per serving: 4 Very Lean Meat.

Preparation time: 30–40 minutes.
Cooking equipment: baking tray.
Oven temperature: 350°F. Barbecue: glowing coals.

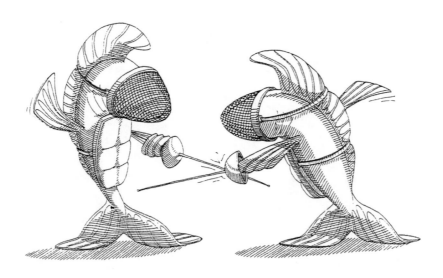

Whole Fish in Ginger

Serves: 4

2 lbs whole fish (e.g.
  snapper or trout), gutted
  and scaled, but with
  head intact
2 tsp chopped ginger
1 clove garlic,
  crushed
¼ cup low-sodium soy
  sauce
juice of 1 lemon
¾ cup dry white wine
4 shallots, sliced
  lengthwise
Garnish: thin slices of
  lemon

1. Using a very sharp knife, score the skin of the fish on each side, three or four times, at equal intervals and at an angle to the backbone.

2. Place fish on its side in a flat dish, or support it upright with wooden skewers.

3. Combine remaining ingredients to make a marinade, and pour over the fish.

4. Bake the fish, uncovered, for 30 minutes or until fish flakes when tested with a fork. Baste frequently with the marinade during cooking.

5. Serve the fish whole with cooking juices and garnished with lemon slices. Accompany with boiled brown rice and a green salad.

Microwave method: At step 4, cover with plastic film and cook on high for 15 minutes.

Nutritional data per serving:
119 Calories, Carbohydrates 1g, Protein 22g, Fat 3g.

Exchanges per serving: 3 Very Lean Meat.

Preparation time: 40 minutes.
Cooking equipment: shallow casserole.
Oven temperature: 350°F.

Vegetable-Stuffed Trout

Serves: 4

4 small trout, gutted (about 8 oz each)
juice of 2 lemons
2 tbsp mixed fresh herbs, chopped (e.g. thyme, parsley, marjoram)
4 shallots, finely chopped
1 tbsp finely chopped celery
2 tbsp finely chopped green bell pepper
4 mushrooms, finely chopped
1 tsp ground black pepper

Serve the trout with plenty of noodles, rice or potatoes, plus a salad, and you have a well-rounded main course.

1. Wash fish.
2. Place each fish on a piece of aluminium foil large enough to wrap it up completely.
3. Pour lemon juice over the outside and inside of fish.
4. Combine all other ingredients in a mixing bowl.
5. Divide into four and pack a quarter of the mixture into the cavity of each fish.
6. Wrap firmly in foil. Seal edges carefully.
7. Bake in oven or under grill until cooked through (approximately 10–15 minutes).

Microwave method: Follow the same method as above except use a suitable large shallow microwave dish, and secure the cavity of each fish with toothpicks. Cover dish with plastic film. Bake on medium-high for 8-12 minutes. Let stand, covered, for 5 minutes before serving.

Nutritional data per serving:
122 Calories, Carbohydrates 1g, Protein 23g, Fat 3g.

Exchanges per serving: 3 Very Lean Meat, $1/4$ Vegetable.

Preparation time: 20 minutes.
Cooking equipment: baking dish.
Oven temperature: 350°F, or use grill.

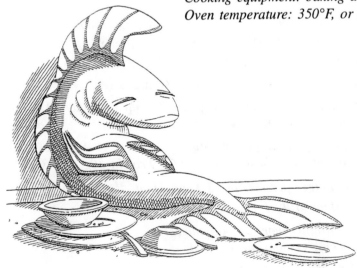

Pasta and Smoked Trout

Serves: 4

8 oz fettucine
1 medium smoked trout
½ cup dry white wine
½ tsp granulated garlic
  or 1 clove, chopped
½ tsp dry mustard
½ quantity White Sauce
  (page 178)
Garnish: 1 tbsp chopped
  capers

1. Boil fettucine in water as directed on the pack, and drain.

2. While pasta is cooking, skin the trout and remove the flesh from the bones by lifting it off with a fork. Break the flesh into bite size pieces.

3. Mix wine, garlic and mustard, and bring to a boil in large saucepan. Add the white sauce and gently reheat.

4. Add the fettucine and mix through, reheating gently.

5. Add the fish, mixing carefully. When the fish is hot, turn it onto a serving dish and sprinkle with capers.

Nutritional data per serving:
356 Calories, Carbohydrates 48g, Protein 28g, Fat 5g.

Exchanges per serving: 4 Very Lean Meat, 3 Starch.

Preparation time: 30-35 minutes, including time for preparing white sauce.
Cooking equipment: 2 large saucepans.

Crab and Zucchini Quiche

Serves: 4

1 quantity Whole Wheat
  Pastry (page 218)
6 oz fresh or canned crab
  meat
1 zucchini, sliced
2 shallots, chopped
¼ cup ricotta cheese
4 eggs
1 cup skim milk
1 cup low-fat yogurt
pepper, to taste
¼ tsp salt (optional)

You can make this dish just as successfully with shrimp in place of the crab, or using fresh seafood instead of canned. Asparagus or mushrooms make a delicious substitute for the zucchini.

1. Roll out pastry and line flan dish. Place crab meat, sliced zucchini and shallots over base of pastry.

2. Blend all other ingredients and pour over filling.

3. Bake 30-45 minutes or until filling is set.

To store: Cover and refrigerate for up to 2 days. Do not reheat or the filling will toughen.

Nutritional data per serving:
654 Calories, Carbohydrates 56g, Protein 30g, Fat 34g.

Exchanges per serving: 3 Lean Meat, 2½ Starch,
½ Skim Milk, 1 Vegetable, 3 Fat.

Preparation time: 45-60 minutes.
Cooking equipment: flan dish.
Oven temperature: 350°F.

Paella

Serves: 8

2 tsp olive oil
2 lbs chicken pieces
  (no wings), skin
  removed
pinch salt and black
  pepper
1 large onion, chopped
2 large tomatoes,
  chopped
1 tsp chopped, crushed
  or minced garlic
$1/4$ tsp saffron powder
2 cups uncooked, long
  grain brown, or
  basmati rice
2 cups water
1 Chicken Stock cube
  (page 80)
1 small green or red
  bell pepper,
  cut into strips
1 cup frozen peas
12 cooked king prawns,
  heads removed,
  shelled and cleaned
  (tails left on)

This is a wonderful dinner party or luncheon dish served with a green salad and crusty whole wheat bread.

1. Heat oil in frying pan.
2. Sprinkle chicken pieces lightly with black pepper and a pinch of salt (optional).
3. Add to frying pan and brown well on all sides. Remove from the frying pan and set aside on a plate.
4. Add onion to pan and brown.
5. Add tomato and garlic, cook until soft.
6. Add saffron and rice. Stir.
7. Pour in water and stock cube, and mix well.
8. Spoon into casserole.
9. Stir bell pepper strips, peas, and chicken pieces into mixture.
10. Cover and cook in a preheated oven until rice is cooked through and liquid absorbed (approximately 1-2 hours).
11. Just before serving, add the prawns and allow to heat through. Serve immediately from the casserole.

Nutritional data per serving:
313 Calories, Carbohydrates 41g, Protein 24g, Fat 5g.

Exchanges per serving: 3 Very Lean Meat, $2^1/2$ Starch, $1/2$ Vegetable, $1/4$ Fat.

Preparation time: 2-3 hours.
Cooking equipment: frying pan, large shallow casserole.
Oven temperature: 400°F.

Mussels à la Grecque

Serves: 4

2 tsp olive oil
2 medium leeks, sliced
3 large peeled tomatoes
  or 15 oz can tomatoes,
  chopped
1 tbsp tomato paste
¼ tsp ground basil
½ tsp ground oregano
ground black pepper, to
  taste
salt, to taste
3 lb mussels in shells,
  scrubbed and beards
  removed

Black mussels are ideal for this recipe. However, it's also excellent with clams or green-lipped mussels.

1. Heat oil in a saucepan and sauté leeks until tender.

2. Add tomatoes, tomato paste, basil, oregano, pepper, and salt (optional).

3. Bring to a boil and add mussels.

4. Cover and cook until shells open (this takes only a few minutes).

5. Serve in bowls with crusty bread.

Nutritional data per serving:
173 Calories, Carbohydrates 6g, Protein 25g, Fat 5g.

Exchanges per serving: 3 Very Lean Meat, 1 Vegetable, ½ Fat.

Preparation time: 15-20 minutes.
Cooking equipment: large saucepan.

Salmon Mornay

Serves: 4

15 oz can salmon
4 shallots, chopped
4 tbsp lemon juice
2 stalks celery, finely
  chopped
2 tbsp freshly grated
  Parmesan cheese
1 quantity Cheese Sauce
  (page 181)
Garnish: 2 hard-boiled
  eggs, chopped

1. Mix salmon, chopped shallots, lemon juice, and celery in casserole.

2. Add Parmesan cheese to sauce and pour over salmon mixture. Mix well.

3. Bake for 30 minutes. Alternatively, cover and microwave on medium for 12-14 minutes, and then let stand, covered, for 5 minutes before serving.

4. Sprinkle with chopped eggs and serve.

Nutritional data per serving:
291 Calories, Carbohydrates 12 g, Protein 32 g, Fat 13 g.

Exchanges per serving: 4 Lean Meat, ½ Vegetable.

Preparation time: 45 minutes.
Cooking equipment: mornay dish or shallow casserole.
Oven temperature: 350°F.

Seafood Cannelloni

Serves: 4

2 tsp olive oil
2 cloves garlic, crushed
2 medium onions, finely
  chopped
$\frac{1}{2}$ cup tomato paste
2 cups water
2 tsp lemon juice
$\frac{1}{2}$ tsp ground thyme
1 tsp ground basil
salt, to taste (optional)
7 oz white fish, minced
5 oz shelled prawns,
  coarsely chopped
3 oz scallops, coarsely
  chopped
$\frac{1}{2}$ cup fresh whole wheat
  breadcrumbs
2 tbsp chopped parsley
2 tbsp dry white wine
ground black pepper, to
  taste
1 egg, lightly beaten
12 lightly cooked
  cannelloni shells (to
  make handling easier)
$\frac{1}{2}$ cup grated low-fat
  Cheddar cheese

This is a recipe for special occasions. For a family meal, you may like to omit scallops and prawns and use 1 lb of minced white fish.

1. Heat oil in frying pan and sauté 1 clove garlic and 1 onion until tender.

2. Add tomato paste, water, lemon juice, $\frac{1}{4}$ teaspoon thyme, $\frac{1}{2}$ teaspoon basil, and salt. Set aside.

3. Combine remaining garlic, onion, thyme, and basil with fish, prawns, scallops, breadcrumbs, parsley, wine, pepper, and egg.

4. Spoon fish mixture into cannelloni shells, and arrange in a shallow casserole.

5. Pour tomato mixture over cannelloni shells and sprinkle with cheese.

6. Bake for 30 minutes until sauce is hot and bubbling.

Nutritional data per serving:
417 Calories, Carbohydrates 40g, Protein 38g, Fat 11g.

Exchanges per serving: 4 Lean Meat, 2 Starch,
1$\frac{1}{4}$ Vegetable.

Preparation time: 1 hour.
Cooking equipment: frying pan, shallow casserole.
Oven temperature: 350°F.

Meats and Poultry

Beef à la Pizzaiola

Serves: 4

1 lb lean fillet mignon
1 tsp oil
1 clove garlic, crushed
½ cup sliced mushrooms
2 large tomatoes, peeled
  and chopped
2 shallots, chopped
4 leaves fresh basil,
  roughly chopped, or
  ¼ tsp dried basil
freshly ground black
  pepper
salt, to taste (optional)
Garnish: shallot

Although fillet mignon is a relatively expensive cut of meat, in this recipe you use only one pound to feed four people. The meat cooks quickly, so there is little shrinkage and as fillet is lean, there is no waste. The recipe will work just as successfully if you use veal, pork, or chicken. Add a few drops of Tabasco sauce if you want to make the sauce more piquant.

1. Cut the meat into thin strips, about ½ inch x 2 inches.

2. Brush oil over the base of a heavy frying pan and heat the pan over medium-high heat.

3. When hot, toss in the meat and stir-fry until well sealed and browned (approximately 2–3 minutes).

4. Set the meat aside on a warm plate and continue as follows. To the hot frying pan add garlic and mushrooms and stir-fry for a further few seconds until mushrooms are lightly cooked.

5. Add the chopped tomatoes, shallots, fresh basil, pepper and salt, and bring to a simmer. Now return the meat to the sauce and simmer for about 5 minutes, or until the meat is cooked and the dish is hot.

6. Finally, spoon the meat and sauce onto a bed of rice or noodles, garnish with shallot, and serve.

To store: Cover and refrigerate for up to three days.

Nutritional data per serving:
170 Calories, Carbohydrates 3g, Protein 28g, Fat 5g.

Exchanges per serving: 4 Lean Meat, ½ Vegetable.

Preparation time: 15 minutes.
Cooking equipment: large saucepan, large frying pan.

Meatloaf
with Spicy Barbecue Sauce

Serves: 4

1 lb lean ground beef
3 slices of whole wheat
  bread, crumbed
1 onion, finely chopped
2 tsp Curry Powder
  (page 191)
1 tbsp chopped parsley
1 egg
½ cup skim or low-fat
  milk

Sauce:

½ cup water
½ cup tomato sauce
¼ cup Worcestershire
  sauce
2 tbsp vinegar
1 tsp instant coffee
juice of 1 lemon
1 tbsp cornstarch
1 tbsp water

This meatloaf cooks in its own luscious dark, piquant sauce.

1. Combine minced steak, bread crumbs, onion, curry powder, parsley, and egg.

2. Stir until mixture is well combined.

3. Add milk and continue stirring until mixture is smooth.

4. Shape meat mixture into a loaf and place in baking dish.

5. Bake in preheated oven for 30 minutes, or microwave, covered, on medium for 20 minutes.

6. Remove from oven or microwave and drain off any fat.

7. In a saucepan, combine all sauce ingredients, except the cornstarch and 1 tablespoon of water, bring slowly to boil, reduce heat and simmer for 5 minutes.

8. Pour sauce over meat and return to oven or microwave.

9. Bake for a further 20-30 minutes, basting frequently with sauce, or microwave on medium for a further 20 minutes.

10. Mix cornstarch and water to a smooth paste. Remove meatloaf to a serving plate and slice.

11. Add cornstarch mixture to the sauce in the baking dish and bring back to the boil, stirring constantly until thickened.

12. Pour thickened sauce over the meatloaf. Serve hot with vegetables or cold with salad.

To store: Keep in airtight container or cover with plastic film in refrigerator for up to two days. You can also freeze it in an airtight container.

Nutritional data per serving:
289 Calories, Carbohydrates 24g, Protein 34g, Fat 7g.

Exchanges per serving: 4 Lean Meat, 1 Starch,
½ Vegetable.

Preparation time: 1 hour.
Cooking equipment: baking dish, medium saucepan.
Oven temperature: 350°F.

Meatballs in Tomato Sauce

Serves: 4

1 lb lean ground beef
1 tbsp chopped parsley
1 tsp curry powder
3 slices whole wheat
  bread, crumbed
1 beaten egg
2½ tsp water
2 medium onions, finely
  chopped
15 oz can tomatoes
1 tbsp tomato paste
½ tsp dried oregano
ground black pepper, to
  taste
Garnish: parsley

All you need to do is make these meatballs, and cook rice, crushed wheat or noodles, make a mixed salad, and you have a perfect meal.

1. Combine beef, parsley, curry, and bread crumbs in a bowl.
2. Add the egg and water to bind the mixture.
3. Roll into 16 equal balls.
4. Place in a baking dish and cook in oven at 350°F for 30 minutes.
5. Heat saucepan with 2 teaspoons of water and lightly cook the onion until translucent, stirring frequently.
6. Add tomatoes, tomato paste, and oregano.
7. Reduce heat and simmer 10 minutes.
8. Add pepper to taste.
9. Pour sauce over meatballs, place in oven and reduce heat to 325°F.
10. Bake for an additional 30 minutes.
11. Serve, garnished with parsley.

Microwave method: Follow Steps 1 to 3 as above. Then preheat a browning dish on high for 6-7 minutes. Place meatballs on browning dish and cook them on high for 4-6 minutes, turning the meatballs three times during cooking process. Remove meatballs to a shallow microwave dish and set aside. Place onions in a bowl and cook them on high until they are translucent. Add tomatoes, tomato paste and oregano to onions. Cook onion mixture on high for 5 minutes. Add pepper, to taste. Pour sauce over meatballs, and cook on medium for a further 15 minutes.

To store: Cover and refrigerate for up to three days.

Nutritional data per serving:
243 Calories, Carbohydrates 13g, Protein 33g, Fat 7g.

Exchanges per serving: 4 Lean Meat, ¾ Starch, 1 Vegetable.

Preparation time: 1½ hours.
Cooking equipment: baking dish, saucepan.
Oven temperature: 350°F then 325°F

Beef Curry

Serves: 4

1 lb lean beef
ground black pepper
2 tsp oil (optional)
1 large onion peeled
  and chopped
2 potatoes scrubbed and
  chopped
½ cup skinned and
  chopped pumpkin
½ cup peeled and
  chopped sweet potato
2 medium zucchini cut into
  chunks
1 tsp dried coriander
1 tsp dried cumin
½ tsp dried cardamom
2 tsp mustard seeds
½–1 tsp dried ground
  chilies
2 tsp finely chopped or
  minced fresh ginger
2 tsp finely chopped or
  minced garlic
1 cup water
pinch of salt, to taste
  (optional)

This dish is best when prepared the day before eating, to allow the flavor to develop. A pinch of salt helps bring out the taste of the spices, but use discretion.

1. Trim any fat from meat. Cut into 1 inch cubes and sprinkle with pepper.

2. In a frying pan, fry (or sauté in 2 tsp of hot oil) until browned on all sides. Set aside in a bowl.

3. In the same frying pan, sauté the vegetables and set aside with the meat.

4. Now add to the frying pan the dry spices and cook for 3-4 minutes over medium heat to release the fragrance, then add the ginger and garlic.

5. Add water and stir the pan juices well.

6. Return meat and vegetables to pan, add salt if desired, and stir to combine the flavors.

7. Spoon into casserole, cover and cook in oven for approximately 1½–2 hours until meat is tender.

8. Serve with brown rice and the accompaniments suggested on page 114.

To store: Cover and refrigerate for up to four days.

Nutritional data per serving:
279 Calories, Carbohydrates 18g, Protein 31g, Fat 9g.

Exchanges per serving: 4 Lean Meat, ½ Vegetable, 1 Starch.

Preparation time: 2½ hours.
Cooking equipment: large frying pan, casserole.
Oven temperature: 400°F.

Curry Accompaniments

For centuries, Indian chefs have complemented the pungent taste of their curries with a soothing side dish. We like Fresh Mango Chutney (page 189), pineapple with raisins, or coconut with diced apple. You will find that the refreshing tastes of any of the following side dishes will also greatly enhance your curry entrée. (Each side dish serves two people.)

Tomato Mint Salad

Mix 2 ripe tomatoes, finely chopped, with 4 shallots sliced and 4 tsp chopped fresh mint. Chill until ready to serve.

Nutrition data per serving: 9 Calories, Carbohydrates 2 g, Protein 1 g, Fat 0 g.

Banana-Yogurt Relish

Slice 4 firm bananas and sprinkle them with 2 tbsp of shredded coconut. Spoon ½ cup of low-fat yogurt over bananas and combine. Chill until ready to serve.

Nutrition data per serving: 93 Calories, Carbohydrates 17 g, Protein 2 g, Fat 2 g.

Cucumber and Yogurt

Combine 2 pieces of cucumber (about 4 inches long each) with 4 tsp lemon juice and 1 tsp of mustard seeds. Spoon ½ cup of low-fat yogurt over the cucumber pieces and combine with yogurt. Chill until ready to serve.

Nutrition data per serving: 11 Calories, Carbohydrates 1 g, Protein 1 g, Fat 0 g.

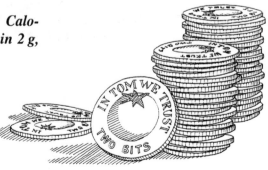

Skewered Lamb

Serves: 4

(3 skewers each)

1 cup low-fat natural
yogurt
3 tbsp French mustard
¼ tsp ground thyme
¼ tsp ground oregano
2 sprigs rosemary
2 bay leaves
1 lb diced lean lamb

*Baked potatoes and a large mixed salad makes this a memorable
meal.*

1. Mix yogurt with mustard and herbs, add lamb, and stir
   well.

2. Stand for 10-12 hours.

3. Remove rosemary and bay leaves.

4. Thread meat onto skewers, grill or barbecue until cooked.

Nutritional data per serving:
178 Calories, Carbohydrates 3g, Protein 30g, Fat 5g.

Exchanges per serving: ¼ Skim Milk, 4 Lean Meat.

Preparation time: 1 hour, plus 10-12 hours marinating time.
*Cooking equipment: 12 wooden skewers (soaked in water for
1 hour before using to prevent burning), grill or barbecue.*

Steak and Black Bean Sauce

Serves: 4

2 tsp oil
1 lb fillet or lean rump
steak, trimmed of fat
1 medium onion, peeled
and quartered
¼ cup coarsely chopped
green bell pepper
¼ cup coarsely chopped
bell pepper
1 medium carrot, cut into
rings
1 quantity Black Bean
Sauce (page 183)

*None of the ingredients in this recipe should be cooked for
more than a few minutes. At the table, the vegetables should
still be crisp and have their true vibrant color.*

1. Brush oil over the base of a frying pan or wok and heat
   over high heat.

2. Slice steak into very thin strips 2-3 inches long and ⅓
   inch wide. Sauté quickly for about 3 minutes.

3. Add vegetables and stir-fry for a further 2 minutes.

4. Add black bean sauce, cover and simmer gently for 5
   minutes.

5. Serve with boiled brown rice.

Nutritional data per serving:
246 Calories, Carbohydrates 6g, Protein 32g, Fat 11g.

*Exchanges per serving: 4 Lean Meat, ½ Fat, ½ Vegetable,
¼ Starch.*

Preparation time: ½ hour.
Cooking equipment: frying pan or wok.

Pickled Beef

Serves: 8

2 lb piece of top round
   beef
12 whole cloves
1 cup wine vinegar (red
   or white)
1 cup red wine
2 tsp brown sugar
½ tsp prepared mustard
½ tsp mustard seeds
½ tsp finely chopped
   garlic
½ tsp peppercorns
1 medium onion,
   chopped

You may never have considered making your own pickled beef, so this delicious recipe may be an eye-opener. The commercial product tends to be full of salt and saltpeter which is not desirable.

1. Trim any fat from meat.

2. Stick cloves into meat, evenly distributed.

3. Place meat in a bowl large enough to hold it snugly.

4. Combine vinegar, wine, sugar, mustard, mustard seeds, garlic, peppercorns, and onions and pour over meat.

5. Cover tightly and refrigerate for three days, turning once or twice each day.

6. Remove meat from bowl and place in large saucepan.

7. Strain marinating liquid through a sieve into smaller saucepan. Bring to boil and strain over meat.

8. Cover, bring to boil, immediately lower the heat and simmer gently until meat is cooked through (about 1 hour).

9. Serve hot with boiled or mashed potatoes and cooked red cabbage, or cold with bread or with a salad.

To store: Cover and refrigerate for up to one week. Excellent to take camping.

Nutritional data per serving:
157 Calories, Carbohydrates 2g, Protein 27g, Fat 5g.

Exchanges per serving: 4 Lean Meat, ½ Vegetable.

Preparation time: 1½ hours plus 3 days marinating.
Cooking equipment: saucepan, large saucepan with lid.

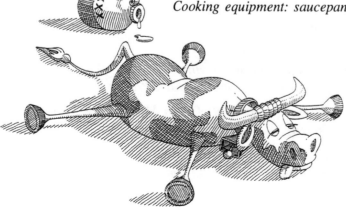

Chili Con Carne

Serves: 4

1 lb top round, cubed
2 tsp oil (optional)
1 large onion, chopped
4 large tomatoes, chopped
5 oz can tomato paste
1 cup water and ¼ cup water
15 oz can red kidney beans
2 tsp Tabasco sauce
¼ tsp ground black pepper
1 tbsp cornstarch

This dish is equally successful if you use lean ground beef instead of top round.

1. Trim off all fat from top round and cut into 1 inch cubes.
2. Brush frying pan with oil and brown meat or fry meat without oil until well browned.
3. Spoon into casserole.
4. Add onion to frying pan and sauté until lightly browned.
5. Add tomatoes and cook over medium heat until soft. Stir occasionally.
6. Stir in tomato paste and 1 cup water. Mix well.
7. Rinse kidney beans, drain well, and add to the mixture.
8. Add Tabasco sauce and pepper, pour over meat and combine.
9. Mix cornstarch with ¼ cup water. When smooth stir into mixture.
10. Cover casserole, cook in oven until meat is tender (approximately 1½ hours).

To store: Cover and refrigerate for up to three days.

Nutritional data per serving:
355 Calories, Carbohydrates 34g, Protein 39g, Fat 7g.

Exchanges per serving: 4 Lean Meat, 3 Vegetable, 1 Starch.

Preparation time: 2 hours.
Cooking equipment: large frying pan or electric frying pan, lidded casserole.
Oven temperature: 350°F.

Leg of Lamb
with Garlic and Mustard

Serves: 8

3½ lb leg of lamb
2 cloves garlic, crushed
1 tsp dried rosemary
2 tbsp low-sodium soy sauce
3 tbsp prepared Dijon mustard
2 tbsp cornstarch
1 cup water
Garnish: sprig of rosemary or mint

1. Trim all fat from the lamb, place the lamb in baking dish.
2. Combine garlic, rosemary, soy sauce, and mustard and spread over leg of lamb.
3. Bake, covered, in a preheated oven until cooked to your taste.
4. Remove leg of lamb from dish and carve.
5. Pour or skim the fat from meat juices.
6. Blend cornstarch with a little water to form a smooth paste, and add to the meat juices.
7. Heat until thickened, stirring constantly to keep the gravy smooth, and pour over slices of lamb. Garnish with sprig of rosemary or mint.

To store: Cover and refrigerate for up to three days.

Nutritional data per serving:
160 Calories, Carbohydrates 2g, Protein 27g, Fat 5g.

Exchanges per serving: 4 Lean Meat.

Preparation time: 1¾–2 hours.
Cooking equipment: baking dish.
Oven temperature: 350°F.

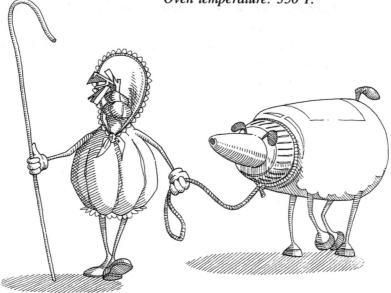

Baked Fillet with Cherry Sauce

Serves: 8

2 lb eye fillet mignon, trimmed of visible fat
2 tsp chopped, fresh oregano or 1 tsp dried
3 small sprigs fresh rosemary or 1 tsp dried
2 cups Cherry Sauce (page 179)
Garnish: 4 sprigs oregano or rosemary

Fillet mignon is an expensive cut, but for a special occasion it is worth it. Remember, too, that there is no waste and, in this recipe, you can serve eight with only two pounds of fillet.

1. Place the beef on a large piece of aluminium foil.
2. Sprinkle with oregano and rosemary, then wrap beef in the foil.
3. Place in a baking dish, bake for 30 minutes in a preheated oven.
4. Open foil and bake for a further 15 minutes.
5. Remove from oven, pour juices into Cherry Sauce. Loosely cover meat with foil and let stand in a warm place.
6. Heat sauce.
7. Cut beef into thick slices and serve topped with Cherry Sauce and garnished with a sprig of oregano or rosemary.

Nutritional data per serving:
174 Calories, Carbohydrates 6g, Protein 27g, Fat 5g.

Exchanges per serving: 4 Lean Meat, 1/3 Fruit.

Preparation time: approximately 1 hour.
Cooking equipment: baking dish.
Oven temperature: 425°F.

Indian Lamb in Spinach Sauce

Serves: 4

6 ripe tomatoes or 14 oz canned tomatoes

1 tbsp polyunsaturated vegetable oil

2 cloves garlic, finely chopped

2 tsp fresh ginger, finely chopped

2 fresh green or red chilies, finely chopped or 1 tsp minced chili paste

salt, to taste

1 lb lean lamb, diced

¼ tsp each of ground cumin, coriander, cinnamon, cloves and turmeric

3 bunches fresh spinach, finely chopped, or 1.5 lb frozen spinach, thawed

1. Blend tomatoes in a food processor.

2. Heat oil in saucepan, add garlic, ginger, chilies, and salt. Cook, stirring, for 2 minutes.

3. Add lamb, mix well, cover and cook over low heat for 30–40 minutes or until lamb is tender.

4. Add tomatoes and cook for a further 10 minutes.

5. Add spices and simmer gently for 10 minutes.

6. Add spinach and simmer for a further 4 minutes.

Nutritional data per serving:
279 Calories, Carbohydrates 17g, Protein 31g, Fat 11g.

Exchanges per serving: 3 Lean Meat, 3 Vegetable, ¾ Fat.

Preparation time: 1½ hours.
Cooking equipment: 1 large, heavy based saucepan with lid.

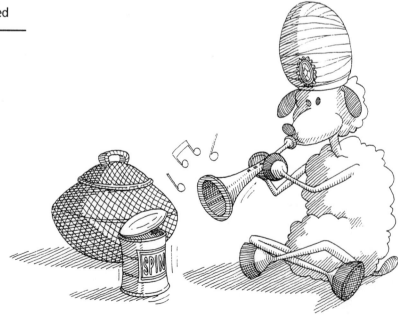

Mogul Lamb

Serves: 6

6 large ripe tomatoes or
  14 oz canned tomatoes,
  chopped
½ cup water
4 cloves garlic, finely
  chopped
2 tsp ginger, finely
  chopped
3 fresh chilies, finely
  chopped
1 tsp ground black
  pepper
½ tsp each of ground
  cardamom, cloves,
  fennel, cinnamon,
  fenugreek
4 tbsp fresh coriander
  leaves, chopped
1 tbsp each of fresh
  basil, dill and mint,
  chopped
salt, to taste
3 lb leg lamb, boned and
  trimmed of all visible
  fat

1. Place tomatoes, garlic, ginger, chilies and pepper into a saucepan and simmer, stirring occasionally for 15 minutes.
2. Add all other ingredients but the lamb, mix well and set aside.
3. Place lamb into a casserole dish, cover well with tomato mixture, cover and stand for 20 minutes in refrigerator to marinate.
4. Place uncovered in oven and bake for 1¼ hours or until cooked.

Variation: use 1½ lb lean diced lamb or fillets and reduce cooking time to ¾ of an hour, or until tender.

Nutritional data per serving:
242 Calories, Carbohydrates 6g, Protein 33g, Fat 9g.

Exchanges per serving: 4 Lean Meat, 1 Vegetable.

Preparation time: 1¾ hours.
Cooking equipment: 1 medium saucepan, 1 large casserole or oven-proof dish.
Oven temperature: 350°F.

Veal Mango

Serves: 4

Sauce:
2 small or 1 large mango
1 cup dry white wine
3 tbsp mango chutney
  or Fresh Mango
  Chutney (page 189)
4 tbsp chopped shallots
Veal:
1 tsp oil
4 lean veal cutlets
2 tbsp water
Garnish: 4 shallots

This is a wonderful recipe that is very easy to prepare and yet looks and tastes good enough for a special occasion. Simple boiled rice and a crisp green salad round out the meal. Pork cutlets or chicken fillets make an excellent and economical substitute for the veal.

1. To make the sauce, peel the mangoes, then cut away and roughly slice the flesh.

2. Place the mango flesh in a saucepan. Add the white wine and chutney. Bring to a boil, reduce heat and simmer until the sauce has reduced by half, about 15 minutes.

3. If you want a smooth sauce, purée the hot fruit mixture in a food processor or blender, or force through a sieve. Return to saucepan.

4. Add the chopped shallots. Return to a boil, reduce heat and simmer for a further 2-3 minutes.

5. While the sauce is simmering, at Step 2, brush a large frying pan with the oil and heat over medium-high heat.

6. Fry the cutlets, turning occasionally, for approximately 10 minutes until browned on both sides.

7. Remove the cooked cutlets from the pan. Add the 2 tablespoons of water to the pan, as well as the sauce. Heat, stirring constantly, for about 3 minutes.

8. Arrange the cutlets on individual dinner plates. Spoon the sauce over and garnish with the whole shallots.

Nutritional data per serving:
245 Calories, Carbohydrates 9g, Protein 28g, Fat 3g.

Exchanges per serving: 4 Lean Meat, $\frac{1}{2}$ Fruit.

Preparation time: 40 minutes.
Cooking equipment: saucepan, frying pan.

Caesar's Chicken

Serves: 4

1¾ lb chicken
1½ cups water
2-3 sprigs fresh dill or
 ¼ tsp dried dill
¼ cup vinegar
1 small leek, thickly
 sliced

Sauce:
7 oz pitted dates
1 chicken stock cube
1 tsp caraway seeds
½ tsp dried coriander
¼ tsp dried cardamom
2 tsp fresh mint,
 chopped
½ tsp finely chopped or
 minced fresh ginger
2 tsp Plum Sauce (page
 190) or commercial
 plum sauce
3 tbsp vinegar
1 cup water

The touch of sweetness and the thickness of the sauce in this Middle Eastern dish come from the addition of dates.

1. Cut chicken into pieces, discarding wings, skin, and fat.
2. Place chicken in saucepan with water, dill, vinegar, and leek.
3. Cover, bring to a boil, immediately turn down the heat and simmer gently for 30 minutes.
4. Chop dates and place in second saucepan. Add stock cube, caraway, coriander, cardamom, mint, ginger, plum sauce, vinegar, and water.
5. Cook, stirring gently until the dates have broken down and the sauce thickens.
6. Lift chicken out of cooking broth, place in casserole or baking dish, pour sauce over, cover with foil and bake for 15-20 minutes.

To store: Cover and refrigerate for up to two days.

Nutritional data per serving:
312 Calories, Carbohydrates 33g, Protein 32g, Fat 6g.

Exchanges per serving: 4 Lean Meat, 2 Fruit.

Preparation time: 1 hour.
Cooking equipment: 2 saucepans, shallow open baking dish or casserole.
Oven temperature: 350°F.

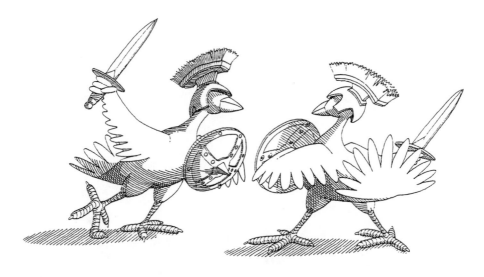

Chicken with Mustard Seed Sauce

Serves: 4

4 chicken fillets, skinless
½ cup tomato sauce
1 tsp Tabasco sauce
2 tbsp seeded mustard
1 tbsp Worcestershire
  sauce
1 tbsp brown vinegar
1 clove garlic crushed

This is so easy to make, and once it's in the oven, you don't need to think about it again until you're ready to bring it to the table.

1. Arrange chicken in casserole.

2. Combine tomato sauce, Tabasco sauce, mustard, Worcestershire sauce, vinegar, and garlic.

3. Pour over chicken.

4. Cover and bake for 45 minutes. Alternatively, cover and microwave on medium for 35 minutes.

5. Serve with cooked rice and hot vegetables or salad.

To store: Cover and refrigerate for up to two days.

Nutritional data per serving:
179 Calories, Carbohydrates 3g, Protein 26g, Fat 7g.

Exchanges per serving: 4 Very Lean Meat, ½ Vegetable.

Preparation time: 1 hour.

Cooking equipment: casserole. Oven temperature: 350°F.

Five-Spice Chicken

Serves: 4

¼ tsp Chinese five-spice powder

½ tsp chili powder (or to taste)

1 tsp low-sodium soy sauce

1 clove garlic, crushed

¾ cup low-fat yogurt

4 chicken breasts (4 oz each)

1. Fold five-spice powder, chili powder, soy sauce, and garlic gently into yogurt.

2. Coat chicken breasts in yogurt mixture and allow to stand at least 4 hours.

3. Place in shallow casserole, cover with lid or aluminum foil, and bake for an hour in a low to moderate oven or until tender, turning occasionally. Alternatively, microwave, covered, on medium for 30 minutes or until tender, turning occasionally during the cooking process.

Note: This recipe is better cooked in a conventional oven than in the microwave.

Nutritional data per serving:
176 Calories, Carbohydrates 4g, Protein 28g, Fat 6g.

Exchanges per serving: 4 Very Lean Meat,
¼ Low-Fat Milk.

Preparation time: 1¼ hrs., plus 4 hrs. marinating time.
Cooking equipment: shallow casserole or baking dish.
Oven temperature: 300°F.

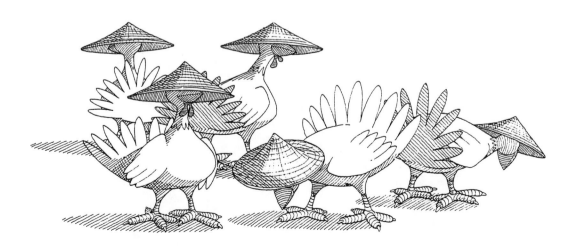

Balinese Spiced Liver

Serves: 4

2 small onions, grated
1 clove garlic, crushed
¼ tsp ground turmeric
½ tsp brown sugar
pinch ground black
  pepper
1 tbsp low-sodium soy
  sauce
1 bay leaf
1 tsp finely chopped
  chili
1 tbsp peanut butter
juice of half a lemon
1 lb chicken livers,
  sliced
1 cup coconut milk
Garnish: 8 wedges of
  tomato, 12 wedges of
  cucumber

Liver—one of the richest sources of iron—should be prepared and eaten the same day.

1. Mix all the ingredients, except the chicken livers and coconut milk, to make a soft paste. It should have the consistency of yogurt. If the paste is too thick, add a little water.

2. In a saucepan, bring the paste to a gentle simmer and cook, stirring frequently, for 5 minutes.

3. Add the chicken livers and cook, stirring gently, until the livers change color.

4. Add the coconut milk and slowly bring the mixture to a boil, stirring constantly. Then reduce heat and simmer for approximately 5 minutes until the mixture thickens.

5. Serve hot on a bed of boiled brown rice. Garnish with wedges of tomato and cucumber.

Nutritional data per serving:
338 Calories, Carbohydrates 7g, Protein 31g, Fat 21g.

Exchanges per serving: 4 Lean Meat, 1 Vegetable, 2 Fat.

Preparation time: 30 minutes.
Cooking equipment: medium-sized saucepan.

Chicken with Strawberry and Peppercorn Sauce

Serves: 4

2 tsp oil
4 chicken fillets (4 oz each)
2 cups Strawberry and Peppercorn Sauce (page 184)
Garnish: 4 whole strawberries

Some unusual combinations don't quite make the mark, but this one is delicious and worthy of a special occasion. You don't have to go to the trouble of fanning the fillets or strawberries in the way we suggest, although this gives a professional touch; you can simply spoon the sauce over the cooked fillets and garnish them with halved strawberries.

1. Brush the frying pan with oil and heat over medium heat. Sauté the chicken fillets until cooked and golden brown. (You can microwave them on 'high' for 3 minutes but they will not brown.)

2. Prepare sauce as on page 184.

3. Slice whole strawberries leaving them joined at base. Fan out from top of strawberry (optional).

4. Slice fillets through and fan across each dinner plate.

5. Pour sauce over and garnish with fanned strawberries.

Variation: Sliced turkey breast with Strawberry and Peppercorn Sauce makes a wonderful Christmas dinner.

Nutritional data per serving:
237 Calories, Carbohydrates 7g, Protein 30g, Fat 8g.

Exchanges per serving: 4 Lean Meat, ½ Fat, ½ Fruit.

Preparation time: 15 minutes (including sauce).
Chicken can be cooked while sauce is reducing.
Cooking equipment: large frying pan.

Apricot Chicken

Serves: 4

2 cups canned apricots,
  packed solid
4 chicken breasts (4 oz
  each)
1 large onion, chopped
coarsely ground black
  pepper, to taste
2 sage leaves, finely
  chopped or ½ tsp
  dried sage
1 sprig thyme, chopped
1 tbsp fruit chutney
1 tbsp cornstarch
2 tbsp water
Garnish: 4 apricot
  halves reserved from
  main quantity,
  1 tbsp finely chopped
  chives or mint

1. Reserve four apricot halves for garnish. Purée remaining apricots in a food processor or blender or press through a sieve.

2. Arrange chicken fillets in a single layer in a casserole. Sprinkle with onion, pepper, and herbs.

3. Combine chutney and apricot purée and pour over the chicken. Bake for 30 minutes.

4. Mix the cornstarch and water to a smooth paste.

5. Remove casserole from oven. Use a slotted spoon to lift out chicken breasts; cover and keep warm.

6. Drain the sauce from the casserole into a saucepan. Add the cornstarch paste to the sauce and heat, stirring constantly, until it thickens. Cook a further 2 minutes.

7. Arrange a chicken breast on each plate and spoon sauce over each one. Garnish with the reserved apricot halves and sprinkle with chopped chives.

Nutritional data per serving:
192 Calories, Carbohydrates 11g, Protein 26g, Fat 5g.
Exchanges per serving: 4 Very Lean Meat, 1 Fruit.

Preparation time: 40 minutes.
Cooking equipment: casserole, saucepan, food processor or blender.
Oven temperature: 350°F.

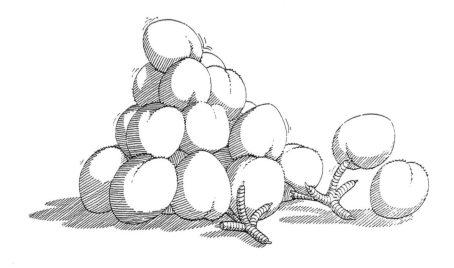

Chicken Tikka

Serves: 4

7 oz low-fat yogurt
juice of 1 lemon
1 tsp finely chopped or minced ginger
1 tsp finely chopped or minced garlic
1/4 tsp dried coriander
1/2 tsp powdered turmeric
2 tbsp chopped fresh mint
1/4 tsp ground black pepper
1/4 tsp garam masala (see Indian Spices inset on page 157)
4 chicken breasts (4 oz each) or thighs (1 lb)

This is simple to make and superbly fragrant. All you need to add are plenty of carbohydrate-rich accompaniments and steamed vegetables or a crisp salad.

1. Combine yogurt, lemon juice, and flavorings in a bowl.
2. Add chicken and cover well with marinade. Cover and refrigerate for 2-3 hours.
3. Preheat oven.
4. Lift chicken from marinade. Place on baking dish. Cover with aluminium foil and bake for 30 minutes.
5. Remove foil, spoon remaining marinade over and bake until chicken is tender and lightly browned (1/2-1 hour).

Nutritional data per serving:
173 Calories, Carbohydrates 4g, Protein 27g, Fat 6g.

Exchanges per serving: 4 Lean Meat, 1/4 Low-Fat Milk.

Preparation time: 2 hours.
Cooking equipment: baking dish.
Oven temperature: 400°F.

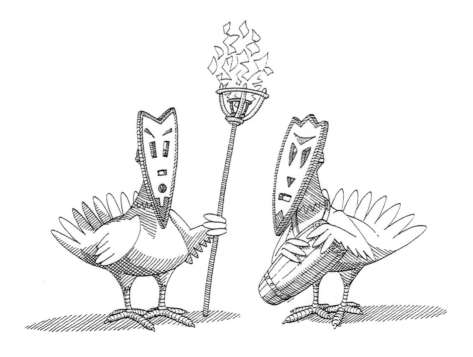

Saté Chicken

Serves: 4

(3 skewers each)

1 lb chicken cutlets
1 clove garlic, crushed
2 tbsp soy sauce
2 tbsp lemon juice
1 small onion, grated
1 tsp oil

A Malaysian recipe that makes a great alternative for the barbecue. Green prawns, pork, beef or lamb fillet are all delicious cooked with this marinade.

1. Cut chicken into small cubes.

2. Thread the chicken onto skewers. Arrange the skewers on a flat dish.

3. Combine remaining ingredients and brush over the chicken. Leave chicken to marinate for at least an hour, turning occasionally.

4. Grill or barbecue the Saté Chicken, turning frequently and basting from time to time with marinade.

5. Serve hot, accompanied by Peanut Sauce (page 179), Gado Gado (page 98) and brown rice.

To store: Use on day of preparation. However, the dish may be made some hours ahead of time and kept, covered, in the refrigerator. You can freeze uncooked saté.

Nutritional data per serving:
169 Calories, Carbohydrates 1g, Protein 26g, Fat 7g.

Exchanges per serving: 4 Very Lean Meat, 1/4 Fat.

Preparation time: 1 1/2 hours (including marinading).
Cooking equipment: 12 wooden skewers, (soak skewers in water for an hour before using to prevent burning) grill or barbecue.

Golden Chicken Risotto

Serves: 4

2 tbsp water
1 large onion, chopped
1 clove garlic, crushed
1½ cups uncooked brown or basmati rice
2½ pints Chicken Stock (page 80) or 4 chicken stock cubes dissolved in 6 cups water
4 chicken breasts (4 oz each), finely diced
1 tsp powdered turmeric
20 almonds, blanched and halved
3 tbsp raisins

There are two ways of preparing this dish—on top of the stove or in the oven. They are equally effective.

Method 1—Preparing risotto on top of the stove:

1. In a large saucepan, heat the water to boiling, add the onion and cook until softened.

2. Add the garlic and cook for 2 minutes.

3. Add the rice and one quarter of the chicken stock. Bring to a boil. Reduce heat and simmer for 20 minutes, stirring occasionally and adding more stock, as necessary, to prevent sticking.

4. Add the diced chicken breasts, turmeric, almonds, and raisins.

5. Continue simmering a further 20-25 minutes, adding remaining stock as necessary, until the rice is tender. There should be no liquid in the finished risotto.

Method 2—Preparing risotto in a casserole:

1. Place all ingredients in a casserole.

2. Cover and cook in a preheated oven for 1 hour, or until rice has absorbed the stock and is tender.

Serve hot, accompanied by a green salad.

Nutritional data per serving:
488 Calories, Carbohydrates 65g, Protein 32g, Fat 11g.

Exchanges per serving: 4 Very Lean Meat, 4 Starch, ⅓ Fruit, 1 Fat.

Preparation time: approximately 1 hour.
Cooking equipment: saucepan, large saucepan or casserole with lid.
Oven temperature: 350°F.

Chicken Enchiladas

Serves: 4

2 cups cooked, chopped
  chicken breast
1 small onion, finely
  chopped
1 ripe avocado
juice ½ lemon
8–10 drops Tabasco
  sauce or according to
  taste
¼ tsp salt
¼ tsp ground black
  pepper
4 small whole wheat pita
  pockets or 8 small flour
  tortillas
2 cups fresh tomato
  purée or commercial
  pasta sauce (meatless)
additional Tabasco sauce,
  to taste
½ cup low-fat Cheddar
  cheese, grated

Don't try storing the enchiladas, they will become soggy. You should serve them as soon as they are heated through. Heat them in the oven, not in the microwave.

1. Combine chicken and onion in mixing bowl.

2. Peel avocado, remove stone. Mash flesh in a separate bowl with lemon juice.

3. Add Tabasco sauce, salt, and pepper and add to chicken mixture.

4. Mix well. Taste and adjust seasoning.

5. Split pita pockets in half so there are eight rounds.

6. Wrap each pita half (or one tortilla) around one eighth of chicken mixture. Pack into casserole or baking dish.

7. Combine tomato purée with Tabasco sauce, and pour tomato purée over chicken rolls.

8. Sprinkle with cheese.

9. Bake in a preheated oven until rolls are heated through and cheese has melted.

Nutritional data per serving:
486 Calories, Carbohydrates 26g, Protein 39g, Fat 25g.

Exchanges per serving: 4 Lean Meat, 2 Starch, 2 Fat, 1 Vegetable.

Preparation time: 1 hour.
Cooking equipment: saucepan, shallow baking dish or casserole.
Oven temperature: 400°F.

Chicken Soy

Serves: 4

4 shallots, chopped

2 cloves garlic, crushed

2 tsp grated green ginger

$\frac{1}{3}$ cup low-sodium soy sauce

3 tbsp dry sherry

4 chicken breasts (4 oz each)

Garnish: chopped parsley, chives or shallots

Try a garnish of three tablespoons of sesame seeds added before baking instead of the garnish suggested in the recipe.

1. Prepare the marinade. In a bowl, combine all the ingredients, except the chicken.

2. Arrange the chicken breasts in a baking dish. Pour the marinade over the chicken breasts. Cover with plastic film and refrigerate for 2 hours, turning occasionally.

3. Bake them, uncovered, for 40 minutes, basting occasionally, or cover and microwave on medium for 20-25 minutes.

4. Remove chicken from baking dish and arrange on a serving platter. Brush with pan juices. Sprinkle with chopped parsley, chives, or shallots.

To store: Cover and refrigerate for up to three days after cooking. Not recommended for freezing as the chicken dries out.

Nutritional data per serving:
164 Calories, Carbohydrates 3g, Protein 26g, Fat 5g.

Exchanges per serving: 4 Very Lean Meat, $\frac{1}{2}$ Vegetable.

Preparation time: 3 hours, including marinating time.
Cooking equipment: baking dish.
Oven temperature: 350°F.

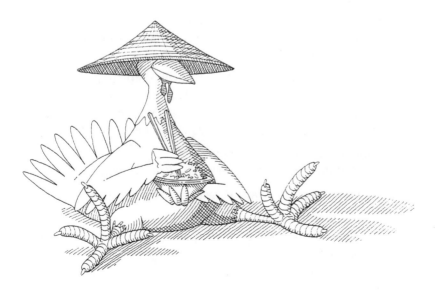

Pork Tango

Serves: 4

1 cup boiling water
½ cup dried apricots
1 tbsp dried currants
1 lb pork tenderloin,
   trimmed of fat
1 beaten egg
2 tsp sesame seeds
2 tbsp fresh bread crumbs
1 clove garlic, finely
   chopped or minced
   (optional)
2 tbsp mango chutney
   or Fresh Mango Chutney
   (page 189)
1 tbsp brandy
¼ cup canned
   evaporated skim milk

This is one of our favorite recipes. The brandy loses its alcohol during heating, but rounds out the lovely fruity sauce. Leave it out if you prefer. You can substitute half a cup of crushed pineapple for the apricots, but remember to reduce the water to half a cup.

1. Pour boiling water over apricots and currants in a bowl, and let stand for half an hour.

2. Roll pork first in egg and then in a mixture of sesame seeds, bread crumbs and garlic until well coated.

3. Place in roasting pan and bake, uncovered, in a preheated oven for 45 minutes.

4. While meat is cooking, heat apricots in a saucepan with the currants and the water in which they were soaked.

5. Simmer gently until water is almost absorbed.

6. Add chutney and brandy and stir until the sauce returns to a simmer.

7. Pour evaporated skim milk in a heat-resistant bowl and gradually stir in the hot apricot mixture (this method will prevent the milk from curdling).

8. Return to saucepan and reheat without boiling.

9. To test if meat is cooked, pierce with a skewer. Juice should be clear.

10. Cut meat into eight slices, arrange two slices on each serving plate and spoon sauce over, distributing apricot halves evenly.

To store: Both meat and sauce will keep for two days if well covered in the refrigerator. They can be served cold, in which case store meat in one piece and slice thinly just before serving, using the cold sauce as an accompaniment.

Nutritional data per serving:
252 Calories, Carbohydrates 22g, Protein 34g, Fat 4g.

Exchanges per serving: 4 Lean Meat, 1½ Fruit.

Preparation time: 1 hour.
Cooking equipment: roasting pan, small saucepan, heat-proof bowl.
Oven temperature: 400°F.

Chinese Stir-fry Pork

Serves: 4-5

1 lb pork tenderloin
1 tbsp polyunsaturated
oil
$\frac{1}{2}$ tsp grated ginger
1 clove garlic, crushed
pinch Chinese five
spice powder
1 cup small broccoli
florets
1 cup small cauliflower
florets
$\frac{1}{2}$ green bell pepper,
diced
2 medium carrots, cut
into matchsticks
3 shallots, chopped
16–20 snow peas
10–12 button
mushrooms, sliced
2 stalks celery sliced
diagonally
1 apple, cut into slices
$\frac{1}{4}$ cucumber, cut into
slices
1 tbsp low-sodium soy sauce
1 tbsp honey
1 tbsp tomato sauce
1$\frac{1}{2}$ tbsp cornstarch
1 cup Chicken Stock
(page 80)

The secret of a successful stir-fry is to have all the ingredients prepared before you begin cooking, and then to cook them swiftly so that they reach the table still crisp and alive with color.

1. Prepare pork by slicing thinly at an angle.

2. Heat oil in pan until very hot. Add pork, ginger, garlic, and five spice. Stir-fry for 3-5 minutes.

3. Add broccoli, cauliflower, bell pepper, and carrots. Stir-fry 1-2 minutes, making sure that nothing is allowed to over-cook and become limp.

4. Now add the rest of the vegetables and continue stir-frying over high heat for another 1-2 minutes.

5. In a bowl, combine soy sauce, honey, tomato sauce, cornstarch, and chicken stock. Add mixture to the pork and vegetables, bring to a boil, cover, turn down the heat and simmer 2-3 minutes only.

6. Serve on a bed of boiled brown rice.

Variation: Replace the pork with chicken or veal.

Nutritional data per serving (based on 4 servings):
318 Calories, Carbohydrates 25g, Protein 31g, Fat 11g.

Exchanges per serving: 4 Lean Meat, 3 Vegetable, $\frac{3}{4}$ Fat,
$\frac{1}{2}$ Fruit.

Preparation time: 45 minutes.
Cooking equipment: large saucepan or wok.

Malaysian Fried Rice Noodles (Char Kway Teow)

Serves: 4

1 tbsp peanut oil
1 clove garlic, finely
  chopped
2 small onions, sliced
1–2 fresh chilies,
  seeded and chopped
3 oz barbecued lean
  pork, cut into strips
5 oz small green prawns,
  shelled and deveined
5 oz calamari (squid) rings
1 cup bean sprouts
10 oz fresh rice noodles
  (kway teow)
2 tbsp low-sodium soy
  sauce
2 tsp oyster sauce
pepper, to taste
2 eggs, beaten
Garnish: 3 shallots,
  chopped

1. Heat ½ oil in wok and fry garlic, onion, and chili until soft.
2. Add pork, prawns, and calamari and continue cooking for 2–3 minutes or until seafood is cooked.
3. Add bean sprouts and toss.
4. Remove mixture from wok.
5. Add remaining oil to wok, heat and then add noodles. Toss gently until heated.
6. Add soy sauce, oyster sauce, and pepper and toss to mix.
7. Add eggs and stir till set.
8. Return seafood mixture to wok, mix in well.
9. Serve hot garnished with chopped shallots.

Note: Chinese grocery stores sell fresh rice noodles as 'sa hor fun.'

Nutritional data per serving:
453 Calories, Carbohydrates 48g, Protein 34g, Fat 14g.

Exchanges per serving: 4 Lean Meat, 3 Starch,
½ Vegetable.

Preparation time: 20 minutes. Cooking Equipment: 1 wok or large saucepan.

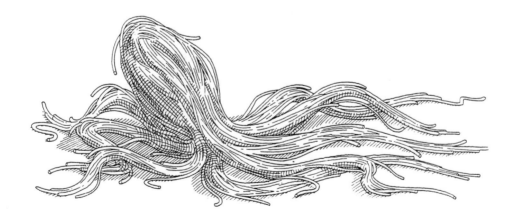

Meatless Main Dishes

Tibetan Pie

Serves: 6

1 quantity Whole Wheat
   Pastry (page 218)
Filling:
6 medium potatoes,
   washed but not peeled,
   cut into large pieces
1 lb frozen spinach
1 large onion, chopped
4 tbsp chopped fresh
   mixed herbs (mint,
   thyme, parsley,
   oregano, marjoram)
$\frac{1}{2}$ tsp coarsely ground
   black pepper
1 tsp salt (optional)
$\frac{1}{4}$ tsp nutmeg
1 tsp curry powder
2 tsp margarine

Keep pastry cool in the refrigerator while preparing the filling; this prevents the pastry from becoming soggy when you add hot filling.

1. Cook spinach in saucepan until excess water has evaporated. The spinach should be fairly dry.

2. Boil potatoes until tender. Drain and mash potatoes roughly so that some pieces remain.

3. Add spinach, onion, herbs, spices, and margarine.

4. Cut off one-third of pastry.

5. Roll out larger piece to cover base and sides of pie dish.

6. Spoon filling onto pastry, brush pastry edge with a little water.

7. Roll out smaller piece of pastry. Place on top of filling. Pierce the top of the pastry with a fork.

8. Trim the pastry to size and pinch the edges of pastry together.

9. Bake for approximately 45 minutes or until lightly browned.

Nutritional data per serving:
424 Calories, Carbohydrates 50g, Protein 12g, Fat 19g.

Exchanges per serving: 3 Starch, 1 Vegetable, 3 Fat.

Preparation time: $1\frac{1}{2}$ hours.
Cooking equipment: 2 saucepans, pie dish.
Oven temperature: 400°F.

Jumping Bean Bake

Serves:

4 as a main course,

8 as a side dish

2 cups dried beans (any
variety) or 4 cups
canned and drained
beans (such as lima,
kidney, or soy)

1 cup tomato purée

$\frac{1}{4}$ tsp cayenne pepper

2 cloves garlic, crushed

1 tsp dried oregano

1 bay leaf

1 lb ripe tomatoes, sliced

2 medium onions, sliced

Topping:

$\frac{1}{2}$ cup fresh whole wheat
breadcrumbs

4 tbsp grated, low-fat
Cheddar cheese

*For a thicker version of this dish, mash half the beans and leave
the rest whole at Step 1 of the method described below.*

1. Place dried beans in a saucepan, cover with water and
   soak overnight (note: do not soak the beans in an aluminum saucepan). Next day, drain the beans and rinse them
   thoroughly in cold water. Return them to the saucepan
   and cover with fresh water. Bring to boil, reduce heat and
   simmer, loosely covered, for 1 hour or until tender: or
   microwave on high or 5 minutes, then medium-low for
   30 minutes or until tender. Drain beans, discarding water.
   If you are using canned beans, drain them and rinse them
   well.

2. In a bowl, combine the tomato purée, cayenne pepper,
   garlic, and herbs.

3. Lightly grease the casserole, and place a layer of beans
   on the base, cover with a layer of tomatoes and then a
   layer of onions. Repeat the layers until all the ingredients
   are used.

4. Pour tomato mixture over, top with bread crumbs and
   cheese.

5. Cover and bake for 1 hour, then remove cover and bake
   for another hour or until beans start to break apart.
   Alternatively, cover and microwave on medium for 45
   minutes, then remove the cover and microwave for another 30 minutes or until the beans start to break apart.

6. Serve immediately.

To store: Cover and refrigerate for up to two days.

Nutritional data per serving (main meal):
382 Calories, Carbohydrates 55g, Protein 29g, Fat 4g.

*Exchanges per serving: 2$\frac{1}{2}$ Very Lean Meat, 3 Starch,
2 Vegetable.*

*Preparation time: 2$\frac{1}{4}$ hours after you have soaked dried
beans overnight.*
Cooking equipment: medium saucepan, deep casserole.
Oven temperature: 350°F.

Vegetable Loaf

This loaf is very high in fiber, and is delicious eaten hot or cold with one of the sauces we recommend.

Serves: 6

2 tbsp water
2 medium onions, chopped
2 sticks celery, chopped
½ green bell pepper, chopped
2 tsp curry powder
½ cup cooked potato, mashed
½ cup cooked pumpkin, mashed
1 cup ricotta cheese
1 cup coarsely ground cashew nuts
½ cup rolled oats
2 tbsp chopped parsley
1 tsp chopped fresh thyme or ½ tsp dried
Garnish: 2 tbsp sesame seeds

1. In a frying pan, heat the water and sauté onions, celery, bell pepper and curry powder for 3 minutes.

2. In a bowl, combine the sautéed vegetables with the rest of the ingredients.

3. Line a loaf tin with foil and spray it with non-stick baking spray.

4. Sprinkle sesame seeds over base of tin, and then shake tin so that seeds adhere to sides as well.

5. Spoon vegetable mixture into the tin and press down firmly and neatly.

6. Bake for 40 minutes.

7. Remove from oven and leave to stand for 5 minutes before turning out. Turn onto serving dish and carefully remove foil.

8. Finally, grill on high for 3-5 minutes or until the top is crisp and well browned.

To serve: Cut loaf into thick slices, but do not separate them, then spoon hot sauce over it (Cheese Sauce, page 181, or Fresh Vegetable Sauce, page 182).

To store: Cover and refrigerate for up to four days.

Nutritional data per serving:
425 Calories, Carbohydrates 25g, Protein 29g, Fat 24g.

Exchanges per serving: 3 High-Fat Meat, 1 Vegetable, 1 Starch.

Preparation time: 1 hour plus preparation time for sauce.
Cooking equipment: frying pan, loaf tin 8 inches × 4 inches.
Oven temperature: 350°F, grill on 'high'.

Vegetarian Lasagna

Serves: 4-6

Sauce:
oil
2 medium onions,
   peeled and chopped
3 large tomatoes,
   chopped
5 oz tomato paste
2 cups water
1–2 tsp crushed or finely
   chopped garlic
1 tsp dried mixed herbs
1/4 tsp each, black
   pepper and salt
26 oz can three-bean
   mix or kidney beans

Layers:
8 oz frozen spinach
9 sheets instant spinach
   or whole wheat lasagne
   noodles
1/2 cup each, cottage
   cheese and grated
   low-fat Cheddar cheese
2 tbsp grated Parmesan
   cheese

This dish is even better if prepared the day before it is to be served, so that the flavor can fully develop. It freezes well, so prepare a few and store them in the freezer as a standby.

1. Wipe a large frying pan with oil. Heat it and sauté onions in frying pan until lightly browned, stirring to prevent burning.

2. Add tomatoes and cook for about 5 minutes, until soft.

3. Add tomato paste and water and mix thoroughly.

4. Add seasonings.

5. Rinse and drain beans and add to frying pan. Combine well.

6. Simmer gently, covered, until you are ready to assemble the lasagne. If sauce becomes too thick, add a little water.

7. Place spinach in saucepan. Cook very gently, uncovered, until it is fairly dry.

To assemble:

8. Spoon a thin layer of tomato and bean sauce over base of lasagna dish.

9. Arrange a layer of noodles on top.

10. Spoon on more sauce, sprinkle with half the low-fat cheese and 1 tbsp of Parmesan.

11. Top with another layer of noodles and cover this with spinach, cottage cheese, and the remaining Parmesan.

12. Place the last layer of noodles over this, cover with the remaining sauce and, lastly, sprinkle with the remaining grated, low-fat cheese.

13. Cover with foil and bake for 30 minutes. Remove the foil, and bake for a further 30 minutes or until noodles are tender.

Nutritional data per serving (to serve 5):
327 Calories, Carbohydrates 42g, Protein 25g, Fat 6g.

Exchanges per serving: 2 1/2 Lean Meat, 2 Vegetable, 2 Starch.

Preparation time: 2 hours.
Cooking equipment: large frying pan, small saucepan, square baking dish.
Oven temperature: 350°F.

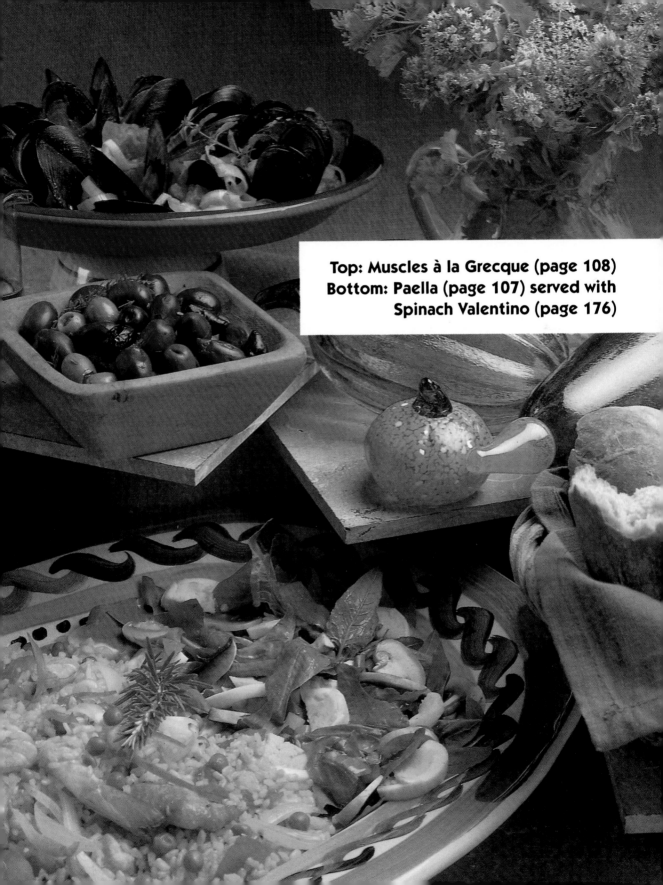

Top: Muscles à la Grecque (page 108)
Bottom: Paella (page 107) served with
Spinach Valentino (page 176)

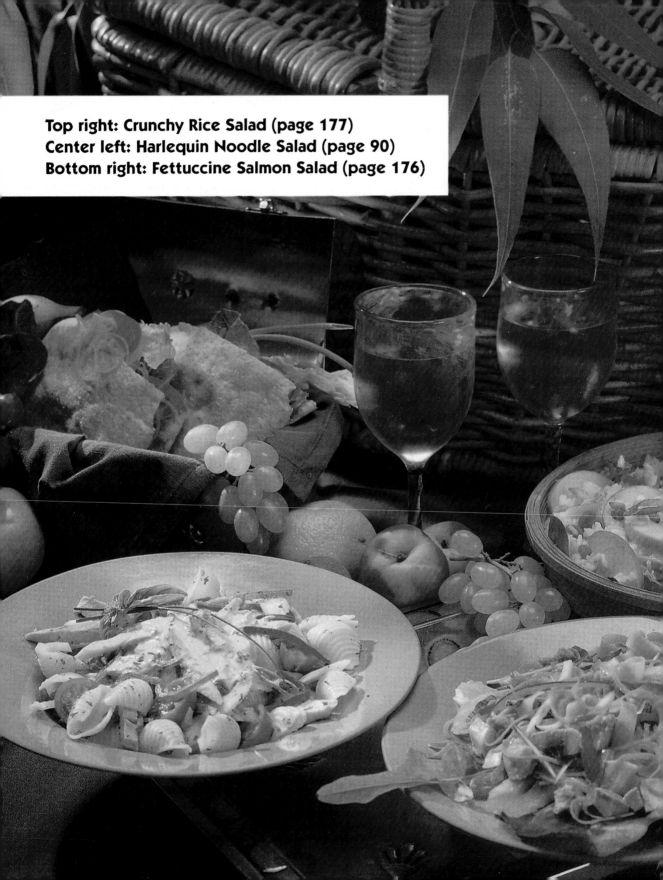

Top right: Crunchy Rice Salad (page 177)
Center left: Harlequin Noodle Salad (page 90)
Bottom right: Fettuccine Salmon Salad (page 176)

Cheese and Spinach Rolls

Serves: 4

1 bunch fresh spinach
   or 8 oz packet frozen
   spinach
2 tbsp water
4 shallots, chopped
1 cup ricotta cheese
1 cup cooked brown rice
2 tbsp lemon juice
pinch nutmeg
12 sheets filo pastry
2 tbsp skim milk

Serve these fragrant rolls with Cheese Sauce (page 181) spooned over them. Try adding 2 tbsp of pine nuts or chopped walnuts to the filling mixture.

1. Wash fresh spinach very thoroughly under cold, running water. Do not dry it. Chop roughly. Place wet, chopped spinach in a large saucepan. Cover and cook over high heat for about 10 minutes or until tender. Remove spinach from saucepan and drain well. Set aside to cool. (If you use frozen spinach, cook it uncovered in a saucepan over low heat until excess water has evaporated; set aside to cool.)

2. Bring water to a boil in a saucepan, add the shallots and cook until softened.

3. Combine onions with spinach, cheese, rice, lemon juice and nutmeg and blend well.

4. Fold a sheet of filo pastry in half widthwise. Brush lightly with milk.

5. Repeat with another two sheets of filo. Place them on top of the first, and brush milk between each sheet. You now have six layers of pastry.

6. Place a quarter of the filling along the edge of the pastry and roll up to encase the filling. Lift and tuck in the ends of the pastry before the last roll. This makes a neat parcel.

7. Place the completed roll, seal-side down, on a lightly greased baking sheet.

8. Repeat Steps 4 to 7 to make four cheese and spinach rolls.

9. Brush each roll with milk. Bake for 15 minutes or until pastry is crisp and golden.

To store: Cover and refrigerate for up to three days. Freezing: do not allow the rolls to brown too much during cooking as they will color further when reheated. Freeze cooked rolls in suitable containers. Thaw completely before reheating.

Preparation time: 45 minutes.

Cooking equipment: medium saucepan, baking sheet.

Oven temperature: 400°F.

Nutritional data per serving:
272 Calories, Carbohydrates 37g, Protein 14g, Fat 7g.

Exchanges per serving: 1 Medium-Fat Meat, 1 Vegetable, 2 Starch.

Spanish Omelette

Serves: 5

2 tsp margarine
3 medium potatoes,
   diced but not peeled
1 large onion, chopped
6 mushrooms, chopped
1 green bell pepper,
   chopped
½ cup cooked vegetables
   (corn, peas, carrots)
½ stick celery, chopped
5 eggs
¼ tsp black pepper
¼ tsp ground nutmeg
1 tsp dried mixed herbs
pinch salt (optional)
2 tsp chopped parsley
few drops Tabasco sauce
   or pinch cayenne
   pepper
¼ cup water

Delicious cold or hot, and is a great way of using up leftover cooked and uncooked vegetables. It also makes a nutritious school or office lunch.

1. Melt margarine in frying pan over medium-high heat.

2. Add potato and onion. Cover and cook over low heat for approximately 15 minutes until potatoes are tender.

3. Add mushrooms, bell pepper, cooked vegetables and celery and cook a further 5 minutes.

4. Beat eggs with seasonings and water.

5. Pour over vegetables in frying pan, cover, and cook over low heat until almost set. Do not allow bottom to burn.

6. Preheat grill to medium, and slide omelette under the grill to complete cooking.

7. Loosen omelette and turn onto warm plate.

8. Cut into wedges to serve.

To store: Cover and refrigerate for up to two days.

Nutritional data per serving:
164 Calories, Carbohydrates 16g, Protein 10g, Fat 7g.

Exchanges per serving: 1 Medium-Fat Meat, 1 Vegetable, ⅔ Starch, ½ Fat.

Preparation time: 45 minutes.
Cooking equipment: large heavy-based frying pan.

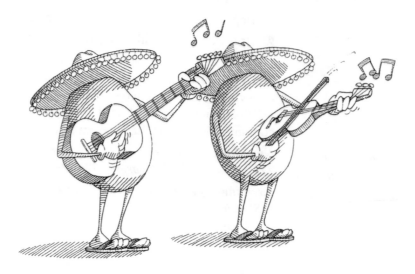

Vegetable Curry

Serves: 4

1 lb mixed vegetables
2 tsp oil
1 onion, sliced
1 tsp ground turmeric
½ tsp ground cumin
¾ in. piece green
  ginger, chopped
2 cloves garlic, chopped
1 or 2 fresh hot chilies
  (optional) or chili
  powder to taste
1 cup water
1 cup coconut milk
1 tbsp lemon juice

Using a variety of vegetables makes this an economical dish based on whatever vegetables are in season. Beans, cabbage, broccoli, cauliflower, pumpkin, sweet potatoes, spinach, potatoes, peas, carrots, eggplant, and zucchini are ideal.

1. Trim vegetables and cut into pieces.
2. Heat oil until very hot in wok or large frying pan.
3. Add onion and spices and toss until onion is golden brown.
4. Add the rest of the vegetables and stir-fry for 2-3 minutes.
5. Add 1 cup of water and cook 6-8 minutes, uncovered, or until vegetables are tender.
6. Add coconut milk and bring to boil.
7. Remove from heat. Add lemon juice.
8. Serve with brown rice.

Nutritional data per serving:
157 Calories, Carbohydrates 8g, Protein 4g, Fat 12g.

Exchanges per serving: 1½ Vegetable, 2 Fat.

Preparation time: 45 minutes.
Cooking equipment: wok or frying pan.

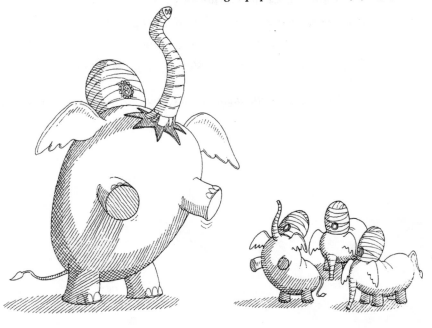

Semolina Gnocchi
with Tomato and Basil Sauce

Serves: 4

1½ cups skim or
  low-fat milk
½ tsp ground nutmeg
1 cup semolina flour
2 eggs
small amount of
  unbleached flour
1 cup of Tomato and
  Basil Sauce (page 180)
  or 1 cup commercial
  tomato-based pasta
  sauce

Gnocchi are best served fresh, but you can refrigerate them for up to three days and then reheat them by dropping them in boiling water. Or prepare the gnocchi to Step 5 then freeze, completing the preparations from Step 6 when you need to serve them.

1. Place milk and nutmeg in medium saucepan and bring to boil. Remove from heat and quickly stir in semolina.
2. Return to heat and stir for 1 minute.
3. Add eggs and work into a smooth dough.
4. Break off small, even-sized pieces about the size of a walnut, roll into balls and toss in a little flour.
5. Half fill a large saucepan with water and bring to a boil.
6. Drop gnocchi into boiling water and cook for about 5 minutes (gnocchi will rise to the top of the water as they cook).
7. Drain. Toss in sauce and serve immediately.

Nutritional data per serving:
257 Calories, Carbohydrates 38g, Protein 12g, Fat 6g.

*Exchanges per serving: ½ Medium-Fat Meat,
⅓ Skim Milk, 2 Starch, ½ Vegetable.*

Preparation time: 30 minutes plus preparation time for sauce.
Cooking equipment: medium saucepan, a large saucepan.

Potato Gnocchi

Serves: 4

1 lb potatoes, peeled, cooked and mashed
½ cup unbleached flour
½ cup whole wheat flour
1 quantity Fresh Vegetable Sauce (page 182)
4 tbsp grated, low-fat Cheddar cheese

You can also prepare gnocchi to Step 3 and then freeze them. When you are ready to use the gnocchi, drop them into boiling water and follow the recipe from Step 4.

1. Half fill saucepan with water and place on stove to boil. A little salt may be added to the cooking water if desired.
2. Mix potato with both flours, then turn onto a floured board and knead gently until smooth.
3. Divide mixture into four, and roll each into a sausage about ¾ inch in diameter. Cut lengths into ¾ inch pieces and drop into boiling water.
4. Boil gently for 8-10 minutes until gnocchi are light and cooked (gnocchi will rise to surface of the water as they cook).
5. Use a slotted spoon to remove onto a serving dish.
6. Toss in sauce, sprinkle with cheese and serve immediately.

Variation: Sprinkle with 4 tbsp chopped lean ham, or use Tomato and Basil Sauce (page 180) instead of Fresh Vegetable Sauce.

Nutritional data per serving:
292 Calories, Carbohydrates 50g, Protein 14g, Fat 4g.

Exchanges per serving: ¼ Lean Meat, 2½ Starch, 2 Vegetable.

Preparation time: 15 minutes plus preparation time for sauce.
Cooking equipment: large saucepan.

Pita Pizza

Serves: 4

4 small whole wheat pita
rounds
1 cup Tomato and Basil
Sauce (page 180)
or 1 cup commercial
pasta sauce
3 large tomatoes, sliced
1 medium green
bell pepper,
seeded and sliced
1 cup sliced mushrooms
1 medium onion, peeled
and sliced
8 tbsp grated, low-fat
Cheddar cheese
oil
16 black olives, chopped
(optional)
1 zucchini, sliced (optional)

The beauty of this recipe is that by using pita bread as the pizza base, you can put the whole dish together very quickly. These pizzas freeze well, making them an ideal snack or light meal.

1. Spread each pita round with sauce. Arrange the vegetables evenly over the top and sprinkle with grated cheese.

2. Place on a lightly oiled baking tray. Bake for 20 minutes or until cheese melts and begins to brown.

3. Serve pita pizzas straight from the oven, accompanied by a Tossed Salad (page 170).

To store: Prepare pizzas in advance up to Step 2, wrap in plastic film or slide into big freezer bags and freeze until needed; then place the frozen pizzas on a baking tray and bake for 25 minutes.

Nutritional data per serving:
335 Calories, Carbohydrates 42g, Protein 17g, Fat 11g.

Exchanges per serving: 1 Lean Meat, 2 Starch, 2 Vegetable.

Preparation time: 30 minutes plus preparation time for sauce.

Cooking equipment: large saucepan, baking tray.

Oven temperature: 350°F.

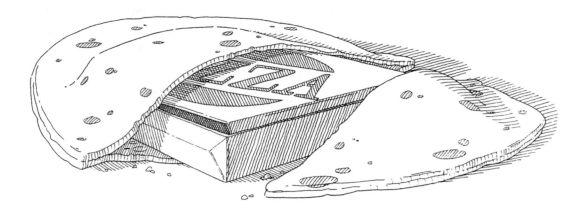

Mexicale Pie
with Cornmeal Dumplings

Serves: 4

2 tsp oil
1 finely chopped onion
2 cloves garlic, crushed
1 green bell pepper, diced
2 tbsp tomato paste
14 oz can whole
  tomatoes
14 oz can corn kernels,
  drained
26 oz can kidney beans,
  drained
½ tsp allspice
1 tsp chili powder or to
  taste
1 bay leaf
2 tsp Worcestershire
  sauce
½ cup water

Cornmeal Dumpling Mixture:

1 cup each, whole wheat
  pastry flour and
  yellow cornmeal
1½ tsp baking powder
½ tsp salt (optional)
¾ cup low-fat milk
2 eggs, lightly beaten
1 cup low-fat Cheddar
  cheese
2 tbsp chopped chives

The dumplings give this already nutritious and flavorsome dish an extra carbohydrate punch. Experiment with the flavorings according to your taste for spicy food. We have suggested canned vegetables and beans to make the dish quick to prepare.

1. Heat oil in the saucepan over medium heat and then sauté onion, garlic, and bell pepper for approximately 3 minutes until just tender.

2. Add tomato paste, vegetables, spices, bay leaf, Worcestershire sauce, and water.

3. Boil uncovered for 15 minutes, then remove bay leaf.

4. Transfer bean mixture to baking dish or casserole.

5. Make the dumplings by combining all the ingredients. Drop spoonfuls of dumpling mixture on top of the bean mixture.

6. Bake, uncovered, for 10 minutes, then reduce heat to 350°F and bake for another 30 minutes. Serve hot.

Nutritional data per serving:
596 Calories, Carbohydrates 103g, Protein 30g, Fat 10g.

Exchanges per serving: 3 Lean Meat, 6 Starch, 2 Vegetable.

Preparation time: 1¼ hours.
Cooking equipment: saucepan, shallow baking dish or casserole.
Oven temperature: 400°F then 350°.

Spinach Fettuccine

Serves: 4

2 bunches fresh spinach
  or 1 lb frozen spinach
8 oz spinach fettuccine
2 tbsp pine nuts
1 tbsp water
1 small onion, finely
  chopped
½ clove garlic, crushed
1 tsp chopped fresh
  basil, or ½ tsp dried
  basil
coarsely ground black
  pepper to taste
8 oz ricotta cheese

This dish should always be eaten freshly prepared.

1. Trim away the roots and woody ends of stems of fresh spinach. Rinse spinach thoroughly in cold, running water, but do not dry. Heat a large saucepan. Put the spinach into the saucepan, cover and cook over medium-high heat for 5-8 minutes or until tender. Remove from heat and drain in a colander. Set aside.

   If you are using frozen spinach, place it in a saucepan and thaw over low-medium heat. Remove from heat, drain well and squeeze to remove excess liquid. Set aside.

2. Fill a large saucepan two-thirds with water, and bring to a rapid boil. Add the fettuccine and boil for 10-12 minutes or until it is *al dente* (tender, but firm to bite). Drain.

3. Meanwhile, in a dry frying pan, brown the pine nuts over medium heat, stirring constantly to ensure even coloring and to prevent burning. Remove from frying pan and set aside.

4. Return frying pan to the heat. Add the tablespoon of water, onion, garlic, basil, and pepper. Cook over low heat until the onion is translucent.

5. In a large saucepan, combine the cooked spinach, pine nuts, ricotta cheese, and the onion mixture. Add the fettuccine, use two forks to gently lift and turn mixture to combine well.

6. Serve hot.

Nutritional data per serving:
376 Calories, Carbohydrates 47g, Protein 20g, Fat 11g.

Exchanges per serving: 1 Medium-Fat Meat, 2½ Starch, 1½ Vegetable, ½ Fat.

Preparation time: 30 minutes.
Cooking equipment: 2 large saucepans, frying pan.

Claytons Quiche

Serves: 4

4 eggs
1 cup skim milk
1 cup full-cream
  natural yogurt
2 tbsp whole wheat flour
1 cup ricotta cheese
½ cup chopped shallots
4 oz mushrooms, sliced
1 medium tomato, diced
oil
11 oz can asparagus,
  drained

This quiche makes its own crust. It is quick and easy to make, and is delicious hot or cold served with crusty bread and green salad. Will keep in the refrigerator for up to three days.

1. Beat together eggs, milk, yogurt, and flour.

2. Add cheese, shallots, mushrooms, and tomato.

3. Pour into a lightly oiled flan dish.

4. Arrange asparagus on top.

5. Bake for 30-35 minutes or until quiche is set and lightly browned.

Nutritional data per serving:
274 Calories, Carbohydrates 15g, Protein 23g, Fat 14g.

Exchanges per serving: 2 Medium-Fat Meat, 2 Vegetable, ½ Low-Fat Milk.

Preparation time: 1 hour. Cooking equipment: flan dish. Oven temperature: 350°F.

Bubble and Squeak

Serves: 4

2 tsp oil
1 medium onion, finely
  sliced
4 cups cooked, mixed
  vegetables (e.g.: potato,
  cabbage, pumpkin,
  carrot, cauliflower,
  broccoli, beans, peas,
  spinach and zucchini)
black pepper, to taste

1. In a frying pan, heat the oil. Add the onion and sauté gently until lightly browned.

2. Add mixed vegetables and pepper. Use a metal spatula to lift and turn mixture until well combined. Then press down vegetables to make a flat cake in the frying pan.

3. Cook over medium heat for 5 minutes, or until the bottom of the cake is well browned.

4. Cut into wedges in the frying pan. Serve brown side up.

Nutritional data per serving:
106 Calories, Carbohydrates 13g, Protein 7g, Fat 3g.

Exchanges per serving: ½ Fat, 2¼ Vegetable.

Preparation time: starting with pre-cooked vegetables, 10 minutes.
Cooking equipment: large frying pan.

Vegetable Side Dishes

Vegetables have tended to become a neglected part of the meal. Yet with a little imagination they can be a feature.

Try mixing vegetables in different combinations, and experiment with adding fresh or dried herbs and seasonings. Nutmeg, curry powder, onion, chives, tomato, garlic, wine, or a sprinkle of toasted sesame seeds or almonds provide a delicious flavor boost. The following ideas may help get you started on a new appreciation of the versatility of vegetables. All the following suggestions are for four people.

Braised Onion

Place 1 cup of water and a chicken stock cube in a saucepan and bring to a boil. Add 4 small, peeled and sliced onions and simmer them for about 8 minutes until they are tender. Lift out the onions and set them aside, add 2 tablespoons of dry white wine to the stock and boil the liquid until it is reduced to about 3 tablespoons. Add the onions, heat through and serve them garnished with chopped chives or parsley.

Braised Lettuce

Wash an iceberg lettuce head and remove any stalks or damaged outside leaves. Cut the lettuce into wedges. Bring 2 cups of chicken stock to a boil, drop in the lettuce wedges and simmer them for 15-20 seconds. Lift them out and, if desired, serve them garnished with finely sliced shallot tops.

Lemon Broccoli

Wash 1 large head of broccoli, removing the woody stem. Cut the broccoli into even florets and steam or boil them for 4-6 minutes until they are tender but still crisp. Drain the broccoli. Alternatively, microwave them on high for 4 minutes. Finally, toss them in a mixture of lemon juice, the rind of 1 lemon and 2 teaspoons of toasted sesame seeds.

Spinach and Shallots

Wash a bunch of fresh spinach under running water. Remove the stalk and chop the spinach finely. Place it in a saucepan with a bunch of chopped shallots, 2 tablespoons of finely chopped parsley, a pinch of nutmeg and 2 tablespoons of water. Cover and cook for 5-6 minutes. Alternatively cover and microwave it on high for 4-5 minutes. Serve immediately.

Diced Parsleyed Potatoes

Scrub 4 medium potatoes and cut them into $\frac{3}{4}$ inch cubes. Drop them into boiling water and simmer them gently for 8-10 minutes until tender. Drain. Alternatively, microwave them on high for 7-8 minutes. Finally, sprinkle them with parsley and toss gently.

Snow Peas and Asparagus

Cut 20 asparagus spears to about the length of the snow peas, discarding the woody ends. Plunge the asparagus (from which you have removed the stalks) into boiling water for 2 minutes until the asparagus spears are tender. Add 20 snow peas, return to a boil and then drain. Make sure that the vegetables don't overcook. Place them on a serving dish and sprinkle them with toasted sesame seeds or almond slivers.

This recipe can be varied by replacing the asparagus with whole green beans or celery strips. These vegetables are microwaved on high for 2-3 minutes.

Succotash (peas, bell peppers, and corn)

Boil or steam 1-$1\frac{1}{2}$ cups each of frozen peas and corn kernels for 4-5 minutes. Drain. Alternatively cover and microwave them on high for 4 minutes. Then add a diced red bell pepper, mix thoroughly, season with freshly ground black pepper and serve.

Pumpkin and Mushrooms

Peel and seed 4 medium pieces of pumpkin and slice each into pieces about $\frac{1}{2}$ inch thick. Place them in a saucepan with 6 sliced mushrooms, a cup of unsweetened tomato juice, a crushed clove of garlic and ground black pepper. Simmer gently for about 15 minutes until the vegetables are tender or, alternatively, place all the ingredients in a microwave dish, cover and microwave on high for 8 minutes.

Zucchini and Carrot Rings

Trim and thickly slice 4 medium zucchini. Cut half a medium carrot into thin rings. Heat 2 teaspoons of oil in a large saucepan, add the carrots and cook, tossing them constantly, for 2 minutes. Add the zucchini and cook, tossing them constantly, for a further 2 minutes. Add $\frac{1}{2}$ cup of water, cover and cook for about 5 minutes until tender. Drain and season with ground black pepper and chopped parsley.

Leek and Apple

Wash and slice a large leek. Peel and slice a large cooking apple. Heat a tablespoon of water in a saucepan, add the leek and apple and toss them to mix. Cover and cook over low heat for approximately 8 minutes until tender. Alternatively, microwave the leek, apple, and water on high for 5 minutes.

Zucchini Creole

Peel and quarter a medium onion, cut half a medium green bell pepper into strips. Place them and 2 tablespoons of water in a saucepan and cook for 2 minutes. Add 4 quartered tomatoes, 4 zucchini cut into wedges, 12 pitted black olives, and $\frac{1}{2}$ teaspoon of chopped fresh basil ($\frac{1}{4}$ tsp dried), cover and simmer gently for 10 minutes.

Scalloped Potatoes

Serves: 4

6 medium potatoes,
  scrubbed
1 cup skim milk
¼ tsp coarsely ground
  black pepper
1 tsp chopped parsley
¼ tsp dried mixed herbs

This is an ideal dish, high in complex carbohydrate. It is wonderfully satisfying just as it is, but lends itself equally to tempting variations. We have given two options, but you can experiment with your own. Although scalloped potatoes are usually eaten hot, they can also be served cold.

1. Slice potatoes finely. Arrange in overlapping rows or circles in a shallow baking dish.

2. Pour skim milk over potatoes and sprinkle with pepper, parsley, and herbs.

3. Bake for 30 minutes or until potatoes are tender and slightly browned on top, or microwave, covered, on high for 20 minutes.

As a side dish: Serve hot with meat, fish, or chicken.

Variation: Omit mixed herbs and sprinkle with sweet paprika, to taste. Or, after the potatoes have been in the oven for 25 minutes, remove them and sprinkle them with grated, low-fat Cheddar cheese, and then return to the oven for 5 minutes or until the topping is golden and bubbling.

To store: Store covered in refrigerator for up to 2 days.

Nutritional data per serving:
135 Calories, Carbohydrates 26g, Protein 7g, Fat trace.

Exchanges per serving: 1½ Starch, ¼ Milk.

Preparation time: 35 minutes.
Cooking equipment: shallow, medium-sized baking dish.
Oven temperature: 350°F.

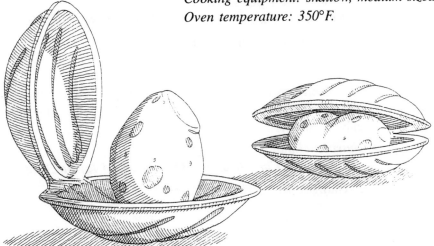

Baked Potatoes

Serves:
4 as a side dish;
2 as a light meal

---

4 medium-sized potatoes
(5 oz. each)

1. Wash potatoes well, do not peel. Prick several times with a fork or skewer. For a crispy skin, do not cover. For a softer skin, wrap potatoes in foil.

2. Bake the potatoes for 45-60 minutes or until tender when tested with a skewer.

Serve plain or try some of the following delicious fillings, or a combination of your own.

Microwave method: Alternatively, wash, prick potatoes with a fork, and cook uncovered in the microwave on high for 12 minutes, turning them over halfway through cooking.

Nutritional date per serving:
154 Calories, Carbohydrates 35g, Protein 3g, Fat 0.1g.

Exchanges per serving: 2 Starch.

Preparation time: 70 minutes.
Cooking equipment: baking tray.
Oven temperature: 350°F.

Cheese and pastrami

Slice tops off potatoes and scoop out flesh, leaving 4 firm shells. Cut 2 small, thin slices of pastrami (1 oz. total) into fine strips and mix with 2 oz grated low-fat Cheddar cheese, the flesh from potatoes, and 2 tbsp low-fat milk. Add a little ground black pepper, spoon back into potato shells, and reheat in oven for about 5-10 minutes.

Nutritional date per serving:
207 Calories, Carbohydrates 35g, Protein 8.8g, Fat 3.6g.

Exchanges per serving: 2 Starch, 3/4 Lean Meat.

Cottage cheese (or yogurt) and chives

Split open tops of potatoes and place 1/2 tbsp cottage cheese or low-fat natural yogurt in each. Sprinkle with chopped chives and serve immediately.

Nutritional date per serving:
160 Calories, Carbohydrates 35g, Protein 4.1g, Fat 0.2g.

Exchanges per serving: 2 Starch, 3/4 Lean Meat.

Tomato and onion

Sauté 1 finely chopped onion in a little water, add 1 medium chopped tomato, ½ tsp chopped fresh basil or oregano and a pinch of ground black pepper. Mix with flesh from potatoes, spoon into potato shells and reheat in oven for 5-10 minutes.

Nutritional date per serving:
167 Calories, Carbohydrates 38g, Protein 3.7g, Fat 0.2g.

Exchanges per serving: 2 Starch, ½ Vegetable.

Spicy yogurt

Combine flesh of potatoes with 2 tbsp low-fat natural yogurt and a pinch each of ground ginger, cinnamon and cloves. Spoon back into potato shells and reheat in oven for 5-10 minutes.

Nutritional date per serving:
159 Calories, Carbohydrates 36g, Protein 3.7g, Fat 0.3g.

Exchanges per serving: 2 Starch.

Duchess Potatoes

Serves: 4

4 medium-sized potatoes
1 egg
1 tsp margarine
white pepper to taste
pinch salt (optional)
Garnish: nutmeg

Preparation time:
  30-40 minutes.
Cooking equipment:
  saucepan, oven tray,
  pastry bag and nozzles.
Oven temperature: 400°F.

1. Wash, peel, and rinse potatoes.
2. Cut into even-sized pieces.
3. Place in small quantity of boiling water and cook until soft (about 20 minutes) or microwave on high covered until soft.
4. Drain and mash potatoes.
5. Beat egg and put aside 1 tsp for glazing.
6. Beat potatoes, margarine, and egg together until fluffy.
7. Season with pepper (and salt, if desired).
8. Fill pastry bag with mixture, and pipe onto an oven tray to form cone shapes.
9. Glaze with remaining egg and sprinkle with nutmeg.
10. Brown in oven for 10 minutes.

Nutritional data per serving:
102 Calories, Carbohydrates 15g, Protein 5g, Fat 2g.

Exchanges per serving: ¼ Medium-Fat Meat, ¼ Fat, 1 Starch.

Curried Brussels Sprouts with Almonds

Serves: 4

20 Brussels sprouts,
   with stems trimmed
   and slit
1 tsp margarine
2 tbsp blanched,
   slivered almonds
2 tsp water
1 small onion, finely
   diced
1 tsp Curry Powder
   (page 191)

1. Drop the Brussels sprouts into a saucepan containing ¾ inches boiling water and boil rapidly for about 5 minutes, or until cooked, but still firm.

2. Dry the saucepan and return to heat.

3. Melt margarine in saucepan, add almonds and toss until lightly browned, remove from pan.

4. Add 2 teaspoons water, onion, and curry powder and stir until onions are lightly cooked.

5. Return sprouts and almonds to saucepan, toss to mix and serve.

Nutritional data per serving:
75 Calories, Carbohydrates 3g, Protein 5g, Fat 5g.

Exchanges per serving: 1 Vegetable, ¾ Fat.

Preparation time: 10 minutes.
Cooking equipment: saucepan.

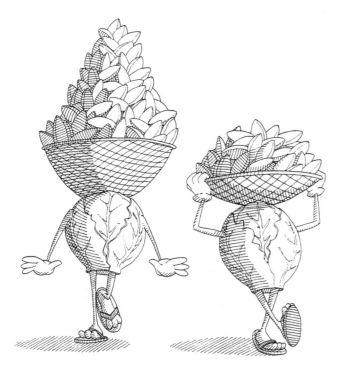

Dry Curry of Potato, Eggplant, and Pea

Serves: 4

1 tbsp ghee or unsalted butter or margarine

1½ tsp panch phora (see inset)

1 large onion, finely chopped

2 tbsp mint, chopped

1 tsp fresh ginger, finely chopped

¼ tsp ground chili

1 tsp ground turmeric

1 lb potatoes, peeled and diced

1 lb eggplant, diced

8 oz frozen or fresh green peas

3 tbsp hot water

1 tsp garam masala (see inset)

1 tbsp lemon juice

salt, to taste (optional)

1. Heat the ghee in a saucepan, and fry the panch phora until seeds start to brown.
2. Add onion, and fry until soft.
3. Add mint, ginger, chili, and turmeric, and stir.
4. Add vegetables and water, mix well and cover.
5. Reduce to a low heat and cook for 20 minutes shaking pan occasionally to toss vegetables and to prevent them from burning.
6. Sprinkle with garam masala, lemon juice, and salt, cover and cook for a further 10 minutes.
7. Serve hot.

Ideal to accompany Indian Lamb in Spinach Sauce (page 120).

Nutritional data per serving:
175 Calories, Carbohydrates 24g, Protein 8g, Fat 5g.

Exchanges per serving: ¾ Fat, 1¼ Starch, 1 Vegetable.

Preparation time: 45 minutes.
Cooking equipment: 1 large saucepan with fitted lid.

Indian Spices

Many spices used in Indian curries are available in large supermarkets as well as in Asian grocery shops.

Panch phora can be purchased pre-mixed. It is a mixture of five different types of seed used whole:

One quantity fenugreek seeds and fennel seeds to double quantity black mustard seeds, cumin seeds, and black cumin seeds.

Garam masala can be purchased pre-mixed. It is a mixture of ground spices which may vary in type and amount.

Some of the ingredients may include coriander, cumin, cardamom, cinnamon, cloves, and nutmeg.

Sweet Potato Patties

Serves: 4

1 lb red sweet potatoes
white pepper, to taste
¼ tsp ground cardamom
¼ tsp ground turmeric
½ tsp finely chopped or
  minced ginger
2 tsp chopped parsley
2 tbsp chopped chives
⅓ cup sesame seeds

1. Peel sweet potatoes and cut into pieces.

2. Place in saucepan (or steamer or microwave) with 1-2 cups water and the cardamom, and cook until tender.

3. Drain, remove the cardamom and mash the potatoes.

4. Add the other spices, ginger, parsley and chives. Then cover and cool (approximately 1 hour).

5. Shape into patties (four large or eight small).

6. Coat with sesame seeds.

7. Place on baking tray, bake for approximately 30 minutes or until sesame seeds are toasted and patties are heated through.

Variation: Replace sesame seed with wheatgerm.

Nutritional data per serving:
167 Calories, Carbohydrates 29g, Protein 7g, Fat 2g.

Exchanges per serving: 2 Starch, ½ Fat (mono).

Preparation time: 2 hours.
Cooking equipment: medium saucepan, baking tray.
Oven temperature: 400°F.

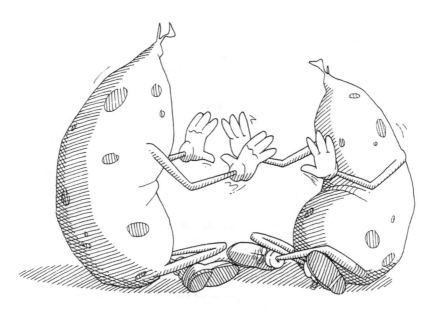

Mushroom and Pecan Rice

Serves: 4

½ cup Chicken Stock
  (page 80)
  or 1 stock cube in ½
  cup water
6 mushrooms, sliced
4 shallots, cut into
  ½ inch lengths
2 tbsp chopped pecan nuts
2 cups cooked brown or
  basmati rice

This filling dish has the complex carbohydrates that diabetics need. It's also wonderfully quick to prepare. Try using walnuts or pine nuts instead of pecan nuts. If you decide to use onions in place of the shallots, then add a tablespoon of chopped parsley as well.

1. Heat chicken stock in large pan or wok.
2. Cook mushrooms and onions in stock for 3-4 minutes.
3. Add nuts and rice, and toss while heating through.
4. Serve hot, or chill and serve cold.

Nutritional data per serving:
183 Calories, Carbohydrates 31g, Protein 4g, Fat 5g.

Exchanges per serving: ½ Vegetable, ½ Fat, 1½ Starch.

Preparation time: 15 minutes.
Cooking equipment: large pan or wok.

Vegeballs

The round vegetables in this simple side dish add an extra dimension to any main course, with both flavor and shape.

Serves: 4

2 tsp margarine
12 small white or pearl
  onions
12 button mushrooms
12 cherry tomatoes
coarsely ground black
  pepper

1. Melt margarine in pan or wok.
2. Add onions and toss gently for 3-4 minutes, until they begin to soften.
3. Add mushrooms and continue tossing until they darken evenly.
4. Add tomatoes and very gently toss until they are heated through.
5. Sprinkle with black pepper and serve immediately.

Variation: Substitute small white or pearl onions with ¾ inch lengths of shallots.

Nutritional data per serving:
37 Calories, Carbohydrates 3g, Protein 2g, Fat 2g.

Exchanges per serving: ½ Fat, 1 Vegetable.

Preparation time: 15 minutes.
Cooking equipment: large frying pan or wok.

Mushroom Stroganoff

Serves: 4

2 tbsp water
2 onions, sliced
1 red or green bell
  pepper, diced
16–20 medium-sized
  button mushrooms,
  sliced
3 shallots, chopped
2 tsp paprika
1 cup low-fat plain yogurt
Garnish: 3 tbsp chopped
  parsley

Serve this dish with brown rice or noodles, or use it as a topping for baked potatoes. It makes an excellent piquant sauce for grilled meats or fillets of chicken and fish.

1. In the frying pan, bring the water to a simmer and add the onion, red or green bell pepper and the mushrooms. Simmer gently for 5 minutes.

2. Add shallots and paprika and simmer gently, stirring occasionally, for a further 5 minutes, or microwave for a further 2 minutes on high. Remove from heat.

3. Place yogurt in a bowl, gradually fold in mushroom mixture. Do not reheat as yogurt will curdle. Garnish.

Nutritional data per serving:
59 Calories, Carbohydrates 8g, Protein 6g, Fat 1g.

Exchanges per serving: $1^{1}/_{4}$ Vegetable, $^{1}/_{3}$ Low-Fat Milk.

Preparation time: 15 minutes.
Cooking equipment: frying pan.

Curried Potatoes and Cauliflower

Serves: 4

1–2 tsp Curry Powder,
  according to taste
  (page 191)
2 medium potatoes (5 oz.
  each), scrubbed and diced
$^{1}/_{2}$ cauliflower head,
  separated into florets
1 bay leaf
1 cup boiling water
Garnish: 2 tsp chopped
  parsley

The flavor of curried food improves with standing, so this dish can be prepared 24 hours in advance and stored, well covered, in the refrigerator. Reheat before serving.

1. Fry the curry powder in the base of large saucepan for 1 minute, stirring constantly.

2. Add all the other ingredients.

3. Cover saucepan and leave to simmer gently for 20 minutes, or until vegetables are tender and the water absorbed. Remove bay leaf. Serve hot, garnished with parsley.

Nutritional data per serving:
91 Calories, Carbohydrates 21g, Protein 3g, Fat trace.

Exchanges per serving: 1 Starch, $^{1}/_{2}$ Vegetable.

Preparation time: 30 minutes.
Cooking equipment: saucepan.

Zucchini and Tomato Bake

Serves: 4

2 tsp margarine or oil
1 round of flat bread
2 medium zucchini cut
    in half, lengthwise,
    and then into strips
3 tomatoes, sliced
4 shallots, chopped
2 tsp mixed fresh herbs
    (e.g. thyme, oregano,
    basil, sage, rosemary),
    chopped, or 1 tsp
    dried
pinch salt (optional)
pinch pepper
$\frac{1}{2}$ medium onion, very
    finely sliced
2 tbsp sesame seeds
Sauce:
1 tbsp tahini paste
juice of $\frac{1}{2}$ lemon
$\frac{1}{4}$ tsp finely chopped or
    minced fresh ginger
$\frac{1}{4}$ tsp prepared mustard
water to blend to a thin
    paste

1. Spread margarine or oil over casserole dish.
2. Place bread in this. Push into corners without breaking it, and leave excess hanging out.
3. Place half of the zucchini in the bottom.
4. Cover with the sliced tomato.
5. Sprinkle shallots, herbs, salt and pepper over.
6. Place the remainder of the zucchini over this, then finely sliced onion.
7. Blend sauce ingredients.
8. Pour sauce mixture over vegetables.
9. Sprinkle with sesame seeds.
10. Fold edges of bread in around the edge of the casserole to form a crust around the edge.
11. Bake for 40-45 minutes or until the bread is brown and crusty, and the zucchini is tender.

Nutritional data per serving:
151 Calories, Carbohydrates 21g, Protein 7g, Fat 4g.

Exchanges per serving: 1 Fat, 1 Starch, 1$\frac{1}{2}$ Vegetable.

Preparation time: 15 minutes.
Cooking equipment: shallow casserole.
Oven temperature: 400°F.

Spiced Rice with Peas

Serves: 4

1 tbsp polyunsaturated
  vegetable oil
1 tsp fresh ginger, finely
  chopped
½ fresh chili, finely
  chopped or ½ tsp
  minced chili paste
¼ tsp black mustard
  seeds
¼ tsp cumin seeds
2 curry leaves
3 cups water
1 cup basmati rice
3 oz frozen peas
2 tsp each of fresh
  coriander, mint, and
  basil, chopped
¼ tsp ground saffron
salt, to taste

1. Heat oil in pan, add ginger, chili, mustard, and cumin seeds and cook, stirring, for 1 minute.

2. Add water, bring to boil and add all other ingredients. Cover and return to boil.

3. Reduce heat and simmer for 15 minutes or until rice is tender.

Suitable to accompany Mogul Lamb (page 121).

Nutritional data per serving:
235 Calories, Carbohydrates 42g, Protein 5g, Fat 5g.

Exchanges per serving: ¾ Fat, 2½ Starch.

Preparation time: 25 minutes.
Cooking equipment: 1 medium saucepan.

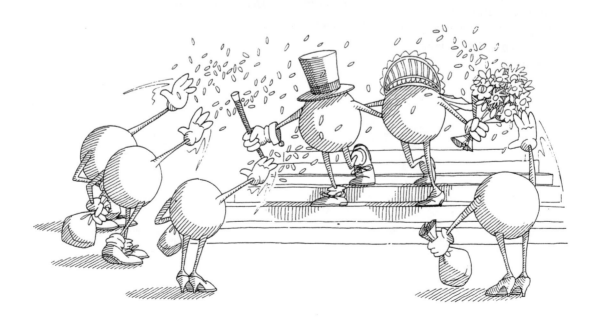

Eggplant Neapolitan

Serves: 4

1 large or 2 small
  eggplant, peeled and
  thinly sliced
4 large tomatoes, sliced
2 onions, sliced
½ tsp mixed dried herbs
ground black pepper, to
  taste
1 clove garlic, crushed
1 cup tomato juice or
  purée

1. Layer vegetables in casserole.

2. Sprinkle with herbs, pepper and garlic and pour tomato juice or purée over.

3. Bake uncovered for 45 minutes.

Nutritional data per serving:
62 Calories, Carbohydrates 11g, Protein 4g, Fat trace.

Exchanges per serving: 2 Vegetable.

Preparation time: 1 hour.
Cooking equipment: deep casserole.
Oven temperature: 350°F.

Vegetables en Brochette

Serves: 4

16 cherry tomatoes
16 pearl onions, peeled
  (or small pieces of onion)
16 button mushrooms,
  stalks trimmed
1 medium green bell
  pepper, cut into ¾ in
  squares
2 tbsp lemon juice
2 tsp low-sodium soy sauce

When you prepare this dish, allow two tomatoes, two onions, two mushrooms and two or three pieces of green bell pepper per skewer. Serve it with brown rice or on a bed of cracked wheat and you have the basis of a delectable meal.

1. Thread vegetables evenly along skewers, leaving about 1 inch of skewer free at each end.

2. Mix lemon juice and soy sauce, and brush mixture over vegetables.

3. Grill for about 5 minutes on each side until vegetables are tender. During grilling, brush with lemon juice and soy sauce mixture at intervals to prevent drying.

4. Serve hot.

Nutritional data per serving:
33 Calories, Carbohydrates 5g, Protein 3g, Fat trace.

Exchanges per serving: 1 Vegetable.

Preparation time: 20 minutes.
Cooking equipment: eight 7 inch skewers.

Orange-Glazed Parsnips

Serves: 4

2 medium parsnips,
  scrubbed and sliced
1 tsp orange zest
½ cup orange juice
2 tsp margarine

Carrots cooked this way are splendid, too.

1. Drop parsnips into boiling water and cook until almost tender (about 5 minutes), or microwave, covered, with 2 tablespoons of water for 3 minutes until almost tender.

2. Drain, add orange zest, juice, and margarine to parsnips.

3. Bring to boil and cook for a further 3 minutes, or microwave, covered, on high for a further 2 minutes.

4. Lift out parsnips and keep warm.

5. Return saucepan to heat and simmer orange sauce to allow it to reduce and thicken.

6. Once sauce has thickened, pour over parsnips, reheat quickly and serve.

Nutritional data per serving:
59 Calories, Carbohydrates 8g, Protein 1g, Fat 2g
(carrot variation: 44 Calories, Carbohydrates 6g,
Protein 1g, Fat 2g).

Exchanges per serving: 1½ Vegetable, ½ Fat.

Preparation time: 15 minutes.
Cooking equipment: saucepan.
Oven temperature: 350°F.

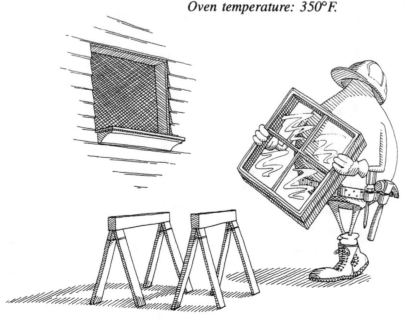

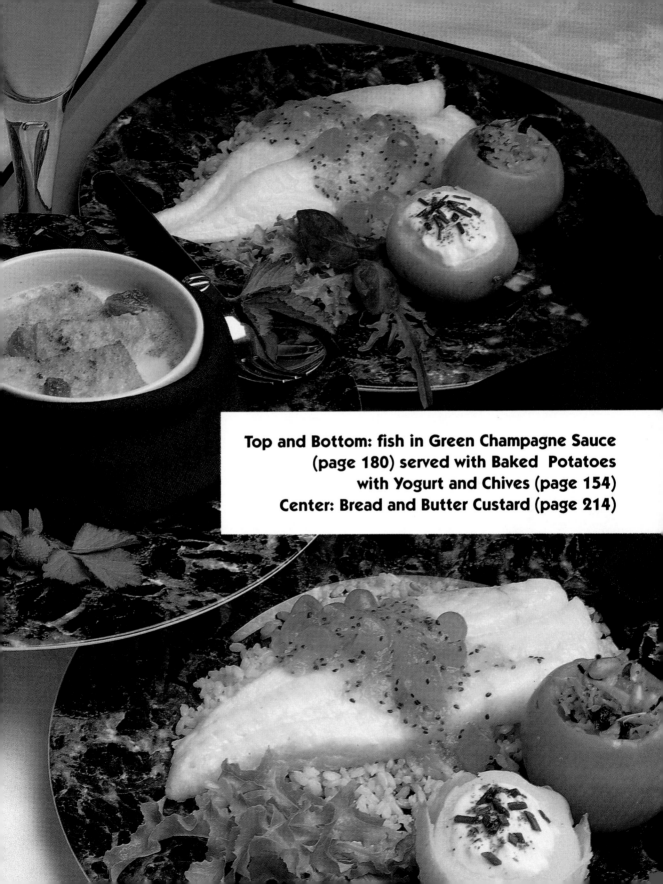

**Top and Bottom: fish in Green Champagne Sauce
(page 180) served with Baked Potatoes
with Yogurt and Chives (page 154)
Center: Bread and Butter Custard (page 214)**

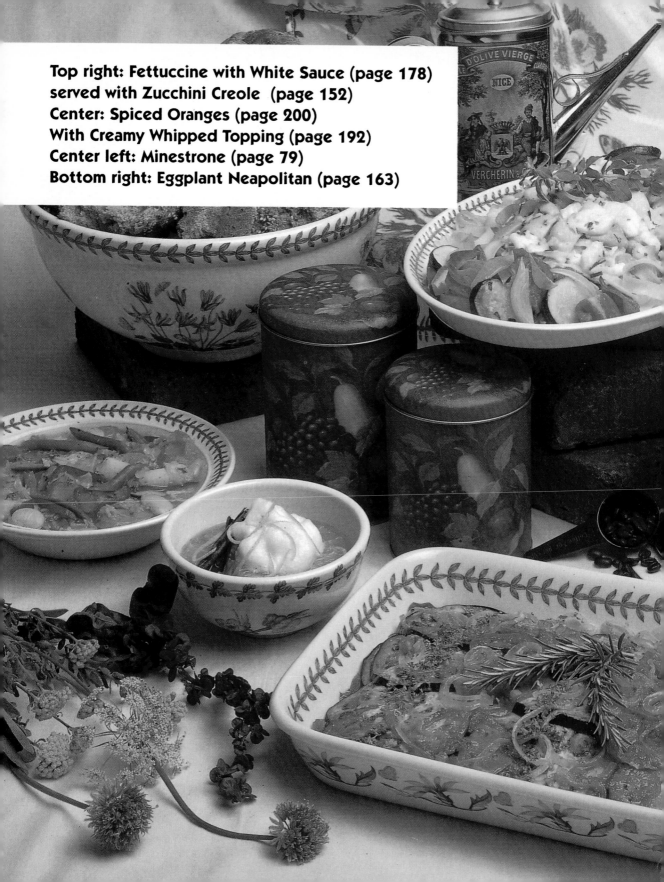

Top right: Fettuccine with White Sauce (page 178)
served with Zucchini Creole (page 152)
Center: Spiced Oranges (page 200)
With Creamy Whipped Topping (page 192)
Center left: Minestrone (page 79)
Bottom right: Eggplant Neapolitan (page 163)

Sweet and Sour Red Cabbage

Serves: 4

1 lb red cabbage, shredded
1 onion, chopped
1 cooking apple, peeled,
    cored, and chopped
1 clove garlic, crushed
1 tbsp vinegar
1 tsp caraway seeds
pepper, to taste
3 tbsp water

This makes a wonderful companion dish to rice, noodles, or potato. Add a small portion of grilled fish or meat and you have the basis for a well-balanced meal.

1. Place cabbage, onion, apple, garlic, vinegar, caraway seeds, and pepper in a saucepan or microwave-proof bowl.

2. Cook over a low heat for 5 minutes, stirring frequently, or microwave on high for 3 minutes.

3. Add the water, bring to a boil and simmer for 10 minutes, or microwave on high for a further 5 minutes.

4. Serve by arranging the cabbage on a hot serving dish, sprinkled with parsley.

Nutritional data per serving:
49 Calories, Carbohydrates 8g, Protein 3g, Fat trace.

Exchanges per serving: 1 Vegetable, $1/4$ Fruit.

Preparation time: 30 minutes.
Cooking equipment: saucepan.

Cracked Wheat

Serves: 4

$1\frac{1}{2}$ cups cracked wheat
$1\frac{1}{2}$ cups Chicken Stock
    (page 80)

In line with the new way to eat, carbohydrate should be central to the meal. Cracked wheat prepared this way is quick and easy. Use it to build a meal just as you would with brown rice or whole wheat noodles.

1. Wash wheat under cold running water.

2. Place in saucepan, pour chicken stock over. Simmer for 10-15 minutes until tender.

Nutritional data per serving:
139 Calories, Carbohydrates 26g, Protein 6g, Fat 1g.

Exchanges per serving: $1\frac{2}{3}$ Starch.

Preparation time: 15 minutes.
Cooking equipment: saucepan.

Crunchy Peasant Rice

Serves: 4

½ bunch spinach
1 tbsp water
1 small onion, chopped
2 cups cooked brown rice
3 tsp low-sodium soy sauce
2 tbsp chopped brazil
  nuts

Almonds or pine nuts are as good in this dish as the Brazil nuts.

1. Wash spinach thoroughly, and cook without any additional water in the saucepan or microwave for about 2 minutes.

2. Drain well and chop coarsely.

3. Heat large pan, add 1 tbsp water and sauté onion until transparent.

4. Toss all ingredients lightly together in pan until heated through.

To store: Cover and refrigerate for up to three days. Reheat before serving or serve cold.

Nutritional data per serving:
226 Calories, Carbohydrates 37g, Protein 6g, Fat 6g.

Exchanges per serving: ½ Vegetable, 2½ Starch, ½ Fat.

Preparation time: 10 minutes.
Cooking equipment: large saucepan or microwave dish, large frying pan.

Hot Shredded Beets

Serves: 4

2 medium red beets
2 tsp margarine
6 shallots, chopped
¼ tsp black pepper
pinch salt (optional)

Beets have a sweetness that adds contrast to a meal.

1. Trim beets, peel and grate.

2. Heat margarine in a frying pan over medium-high heat, and add beets, shallots, black pepper, and salt.

3. Sauté gently, turning from time to time, for about 10 minutes or until cooked through. Serve hot.

Nutritional data per serving:
53 Calories, Carbohydrates 7g, Protein 2g, Fat 2g.

Exchanges per serving: 1 Vegetable, ½ Fat (poly).

Preparation time: 20 minutes.
Cooking equipment: frying pan.

Vegetables Julienne

Serves: 4

1 small zucchini
2 medium carrots
8 French beans
1 stick celery
½ green bell pepper
4 shallots
1½ cups water
1 chicken stock cube

Prepare the vegetables neatly using a small sharp knife. Cook them quickly and serve them right away.

1. Trim top from zucchini. Cut in half, across, then in half lengthwise and, finally, into julienne strips.

2. Peel carrots, cut as for zucchini. Trim beans. Cut each in half, across, then in half lengthwise.

3. Cut celery into lengths, then into strips. Cut bell pepper into strips, removing any pith and seeds.

4. Trim shallots, cut into lengths, then each length in half.

5. Add water and stock cube to saucepan, bring to boil.

6. Add carrots, cook 2-3 minutes, then beans, celery and zucchini and cook a further minute.

7. Lastly, add bell pepper and shallots and cook a further minute.

8. Drain, then gently lift vegetables from water, using tongs or a slotted spoon to avoid breaking strips.

Nutritional data per serving:
35 Calories, Carbohydrates 6g, Protein 2g, Fat trace.

Exchanges per serving: 1¼ Vegetable.

Preparation time: 20 minutes.
Cooking equipment: saucepan.

Stir-fried Vegetables

Serves 4

½ Chinese cabbage
   or ⅛ green cabbage
1 tsp oil
1 small white onion,
   quartered
1 tsp chopped ginger
¾ cup broccoli florets
1 small carrot, sliced
   finely
10–12 snow peas
¾ cup bean sprouts
½ green bell pepper,
   diced
3 oz mushrooms, sliced
½ cup water
1 bouillon cube
1 tbsp low-sodium soy
   sauce

Stir-fried vegetables should be crisp and fresh-colored—the result of swift cooking over high heat.

1. Prepare the Chinese cabbage by cutting off the woody ends of stalks. Discard. Cut the stalks into 1 inch lengths and shred the leaves. Cut the cabbage leaves into shreds about 2 inches long.

2. Place wok or heavy frying pan over high heat. Coat thinly with the oil. When very hot add fresh ginger and onion. Stir-fry for 2-3 minutes.

3. Add remaining vegetables, stir-fry for 2-3 minutes more.

4. Dissolve the stock cube in water, then add to vegetables.

5. Turn the heat down, add the soy sauce and combine with the vegetables. Cover the wok or pan, and simmer vegetables for 3-4 minutes. Serve hot.

Nutritional data per serving:
41 Calories, Carbohydrates 6g, Protein 4g, Fat 1g.

Exchanges per serving: 1¼ Vegetable, ¼ Fat.

Preparation time: 20 minutes.
Cooking equipment: wok or heavy frying pan.

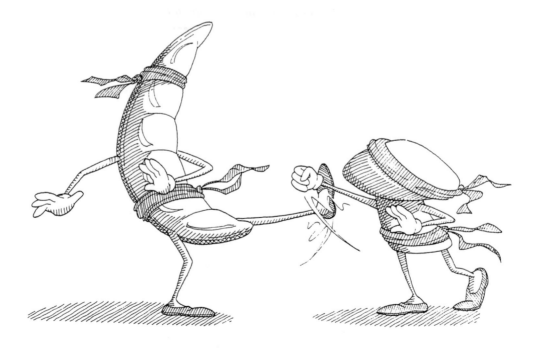

Salads

All the salad ideas we give here are simple, but show you that with a little inspiration a salad can add something special to a meal. All these recipes will serve four.

Asparagus and Green Bean Salad

Trim 8 spears of fresh asparagus and cut them into 3 inch lengths. Trim and halve 12 green beans. Boil, steam or microwave them until just tender, then drop them into icy water to cool them quickly. This helps retain their crispness and color. Drain. Wash and dry a head of romaine lettuce, tear it into pieces and line a salad bowl. Combine the asparagus, beans, and 16 cherry tomatoes and place them in the salad bowl. Pour over ¼ cup of Italian Dressing (page 186) and sprinkle 2 tablespoons of toasted sesame seeds over.

Ginger Carrots

Slice 2 medium carrots into long strips with a potato peeler. Add a little peeled and finely chopped fresh ginger and then pour ½ cup of vinegar over. Refrigerate for 2 hours before serving. You can add thinly sliced cucumber if you like.

Tomato and Onion

Slice 3 firm, ripe tomatoes, and a white onion. Pour ½ cup of red wine vinegar over. Add freshly ground black pepper. Refrigerate for at least ½ hour before serving.

Orange and Cucumber Salad

Peel and slice 2 oranges, removing all pith. Slice ½ cucumber and a small onion. Break the onion into separate rings. Mix and sprinkle them with a tablespoon of chopped parsley and, finally, pour over one quantity of Creamy Orange Dressing (page 187). Chill well before serving.

Mushroom Salad

Slice 10 medium mushrooms into a bowl. Add a cup of bean sprouts, ½ cup each of celery and red bell pepper, cut into matchsticks, and 2 chopped spring onions. Toss with ½ quantity of Orange and Soy Dressing (page 187) or Herbed Tomato Dressing (page 186) and chill well.

Avocado, Spinach and Tofu Salad

Wash a bunch of spinach, remove the stalks and tear the leaves into bite-sized pieces. Place spinach in a bowl and add a sliced medium avocado, 8 pitted and quartered black olives, and 8 oz firm tofu (soybean curd) cut into small cubes. Make a dressing of 2 teaspoons of olive oil, 1 tablespoon lemon juice, and a crushed clove of garlic, pour it over the salad and toss lightly. Chill.

Broccoli, Bean Sprouts, and Snowpeas with Lemon

Blanch 2 cups broccoli florets by cooking them in boiling water or steaming them for 3 minutes. Plunge quickly under cold water to cool. Steam 12-15 (5 oz) snowpeas for 1-2 minutes and cool quickly under cold water. Rinse 1 cup of bean sprouts and combine them with the broccoli and snowpeas in a bowl. Pour over a dressing made of 2 tablespoons of lemon juice, ½ teaspoon of coarsely ground black pepper and 2 teaspoons of oil. Serve chilled.

Tossed Salad

Use your imagination in creating tossed salads. For instance, consider blanched green beans, zucchini, broccoli florets, and cauliflower. You can combine alfalfa sprouts, mushrooms, snowpeas, sugar peas, carrot and celery with the more traditional ingredients such as various kinds of lettuce, bell peppers, cucumbers, and tomatoes. Avocado adds a certain richness. Toss with ¼ cup Italian Dressing (page 186) or a commercial no-oil dressing.

Fruity Noodle Salad

Serves: 4

2½ cups cooked pasta
½ cup raisins
1 stick celery, diced
3 shallots, chopped
1 green apple, cored
  and diced
4 dried apricots, chopped
4 dried peaches, chopped
⅓ cup pine nuts

Dressing:

½ cup orange juice
1 clove garlic, crushed
1 tsp minced ginger
1 tsp lemon juice
1 packet Equal or
  other sweetener
  equivalent to 2 tsp
  sugar

1. Combine all ingredients, except the pine nuts, in salad bowl.
2. Toast pine nuts until golden brown in a moderate oven for 5-8 minutes. Cool and then add to other ingredients.
3. Combine the dressing ingredients in a screw top jar, shake well and pour over salad.
4. Toss salad, cover and refrigerate for several hours before serving.

To store: Keep in airtight container in refrigerator for up to three days.

Nutritional data per serving:
327 Calories, Carbohydrates 56g, Protein 9g, Fat 8g.

Exchanges per serving: 2 Starch, 1¾ Fruit, 1½ Fat.

Preparation time: 15 minutes.
Cooking equipment: baking tray.
Oven temperature: 350°F.

Curried Pasta Salad

Serves: 4

1½ cups uncooked shell
    pasta
½ cup diced celery
4 shallots, chopped
2 tbsp raisins
½ green bell pepper,
    diced
2 tbsp chopped parsley
½ cup corn kernels
Dressing:
½ quantity Curry
    Dressing (page 187)

1. Cook noodles in boiling water for 10-12 minutes until *al dente* (tender), drain and then run cold water over to cool them.

2. Combine pasta, celery, shallots, raisins, bell pepper, parsley, and corn.

3. Toss in curry dressing.

4. Refrigerate for 1 hour before serving.

To store: Keep in airtight container in refrigerator and store for up to two days.

Nutritional data per serving:
133 Calories, Carbohydrates 26g, Protein 5g, Fat 1g.

Exchanges per serving: 1¼ Starch, ½ Fruit.

Preparation time: 1¼ hours. Cooking equipment: saucepan.

New Potato Salad

Serves: 4

16 small new potatoes
    (1 lb)
2–3 tbsp fresh mint,
    chopped
2 tbsp chopped fresh
    chives or 2 tbsp
    chopped shallots
7 oz low-fat yogurt
½ tsp minced green
    ginger
½ tsp minced garlic
½ tsp prepared mild
    mustard
1 tsp lemon juice

1. Scrub potatoes if necessary, but do not peel.

2. Boil, steam or microwave the potatoes until tender. Drain and cool.

3. Place in serving bowl and add mint, and chives or shallots.

4. In a small mixing bowl combine yogurt, ginger, garlic, mustard, and lemon juice. Mix well.

5. Pour over potatoes. Mix well. Cover and refrigerate until ready to serve.

Nutritional data per serving:
155 Calories, Carbohydrates 32g, Protein 5g, Fat 1g.

Exchanges per serving: 2 Starch, ¼ Low-Fat Milk.

Preparation time: 2¾ hours including cooling time.
Cooking equipment: medium saucepan.

Curried Sweet Potato and Banana Salad

Serves: 4

3 medium sweet potatoes, peeled
2 medium bananas
1 tbsp lemon juice
2 shallots, chopped
1 quantity Curry Dressing (page 187)

1. Cut sweet potatoes into ¾ inch cubes.
2. Place in a large saucepan and barely cover with cold water. Bring to a boil, reduce heat and simmer for about 10-12 minutes, or until potato is cooked through, but still holds it shape. Alternatively, microwave on high for 5-6 minutes.
3. Meanwhile, slice banana and toss in lemon juice.
4. Drain the cooked potato and allow to cool.
5. In a salad bowl place the potato, banana, shallots, and dressing and toss gently to combine.

Nutritional data per serving:
125 Calories, Carbohydrates 26g, Protein 4g, Fat 1g.

Exchanges per serving: 1⅓ Starch, ½ Fruit.

Preparation time: 20 minutes.
Cooking equipment: large saucepan.

Tabbouleh

Serves: 4

½ cup cracked wheat
2 large ripe tomatoes, skinned and finely chopped
1 small onion, finely chopped
1 cup chopped parsley
ground black pepper
2 tsp olive oil
2 tbsp lemon juice
1 tbsp finely chopped mint

1. Place cracked wheat in a deep bowl, cover with boiling water and allow to stand for 2 hours.
2. Drain well by squeezing in a clean muslin cloth or tea towel, and return to bowl.
3. Add the tomatoes, onion, parsley, pepper, oil, lemon juice, and mint.
4. Combine well and chill for 1 hour before serving.

Nutritional data per serving:
112 Calories, Carbohydrates 17g, Protein 4g, Fat 3g.

Exchanges per serving: ¾ Starch, ¾ Vegetable, ½ Fat.

Preparation time: soaking cracked wheat 2 hours, preparation 15 minutes, chiling time 1 hour.

Tangy Potato Salad

Serves: 4

3 medium potatoes
4 shallots, chopped
3 eggs, hardboiled and sliced
½ cup low-fat yogurt
½ tsp black pepper coarsely ground
2 tsp Curry Powder (page 191)
4 lettuce cups

This salad is best when made in advance; the flavor develops during refrigeration.

1. Peel potatoes.
2. Cook until slightly soft, but do not overcook as potato will not hold its shape. Drain.
3. Cut potato into cubes and mix with spring onion.
4. Add eggs.
5. Combine yogurt, pepper, and curry powder. Spoon over the potato mixture and toss gently.
6. Store in airtight container in refrigerator until required.
7. Serve in lettuce cups.

To store: Cover and refrigerate for up to two days.

Nutritional data per serving:
131 Calories, Carbohydrates 14g, Protein 9g, Fat 4g.

Exchanges per serving: 1 Medium-Fat Meat, 1 Starch.

Preparation time: 30 minutes.
Cooking equipment: saucepan.

Raita

Serves: 4

¼ cucumber
pinch of salt
1 medium tomato
1 small onion
7 oz low-fat yogurt
pepper, to taste
¼ tsp minced garlic
3–4 drops Tabasco sauce

1. Peel and chop the cucumber. Sprinkle with salt. Place in colander over bowl and allow to drain for 30 minutes.
2. Chop tomato and place in the second bowl.
3. Slice onion very finely.
4. Mix tomato, onion, and cucumber.
5. Mix yogurt, pepper, garlic, and Tabasco or chili sauce.
6. Pour yogurt mixture over vegetables, mix well, and refrigerate for an hour.

Nutritional data per serving:
42 Calories, Carbohydrates 6g, Protein 3g, Fat 1g.

Exchanges per serving: ½ Vegetable, ¼ Low-Fat Milk.

Preparation time: 2 hours.

Coleslaw

Serves: 4

¼ medium cabbage,
    finely shredded
1 small onion, grated
1 small green bell pepper,
    chopped
1 stick celery, chopped
⅓ cup grated carrot
ground black pepper
½ quantity Creamy
    Yogurt Dressing
    (page 188)

Once you have added the dressing, coleslaw should not be stored. However, you can prepare the vegetables in advance and store them in the refrigerator. Add the dressing just before serving.

Toss all ingredients in a large bowl, chill until ready to serve.

Variation: Add ⅓ cup chopped pineapple and 2 tablespoons of raisins. Substitute commercial low-oil coleslaw dressing for Creamy Yogurt Dressing.

To store: Cover and refrigerate for no more than a day.

Nutritional data per serving:
29 Calories, Carbohydrates 5g, Protein 2g, Fat trace.

Exchanges per serving: 1 Vegetable.

Preparation time: 10 minutes.

Broad Bean
and Smoked Salmon Salad

Serves: 4

8 oz fava or lima beans,
    frozen or fresh
3 oz smoked salmon,
    thinly sliced
12 cherry tomatoes
1 small white onion,
    thinly sliced
2 tbsp lemon juice
2 tsp olive oil
2 tsp capers, drained
2 tsp chopped fresh
    parsley

1. Cook beans until they are soft, but still retain their shape.
2. Combine cooked beans, smoked salmon, cherry tomatoes, and white onion in a bowl.
3. Blend all the other ingredients in a screw top jar and pour over the salad.
4. Chill and serve.

Nutritional data per serving:
152 Calories, Carbohydrates 17g, Protein 11g, Fat 5g.

Exchanges per serving: 1 Very Lean Meat, 1 Starch,
¼ Vegetable, ½ Fat.

Preparation time: 20 minutes.
Cooking equipment: saucepan.

Fettuccine Salmon Salad

Serves: 4

4 cups water
8 oz fresh spinach
  fettuccine
6 shallots
½ stick celery
½ bell pepper
1 tomato
½ zucchini
½ avocado
7 oz can red salmon
1 cup grated carrot
Dressing:
2 tbsp chopped mint
juice of ½ lemon
juice of 1 orange
2 tsp olive oil
2 tsp low-sodium soy sauce

1. Heat water until boiling.
2. Add fettuccine and cook until *al dente* (tender).
3. Drain, rinse, and cool.
4. Chop shallots, celery, bell pepper, and tomato.
5. Cut zucchini into fine strips.
6. Peel avocado, discard stone, chop roughly.
7. Drain salmon, remove bones and skin.
8. Combine pasta with all other ingredients and mix gently.
9. Mix dressing ingredients and pour over. Serve.

Nutritional data per serving:
284 Calories, Carbohydrates 25g, Protein 16g, Fat 13g.

Exchanges per serving: 2 Very Lean Meat, 1 Vegetable, 2 Fat, 1½ Starch.

Preparation time: 45 minutes. Cooking equipment: saucepan.

Spinach Valentino

Serves: 4

1 bunch spinach
4 mushrooms, sliced
2 shallots, sliced
2 eggs, hardboiled
1 quantity Orange and
  Soy Dressing (page 187)

1. Wash spinach thoroughly, and shake gently to remove excess water. Remove the stalks and tear into bite-size pieces.
2. Combine spinach, mushrooms, shallots, and sliced eggs and toss in dressing.
3. Chill before serving.

Nutritional data per serving:
63 Calories, Carbohydrates 2g, Protein 5g, Fat 4g.

Exchanges per serving: ½ Medium-Fat Meat, ¾ Vegetable.

Preparation time: 5 minutes.

Crunchy Rice Salad

Serves: 4

2 cups cooked brown rice
½ green bell pepper, chopped
½ red bell pepper, chopped
4 shallots, sliced
4 radishes, finely sliced
1 stick celery, finely sliced
¼ cup unsalted, roasted peanuts
½ cup canned water chestnuts, drained and sliced
½ cup green beans, lightly cooked
1 tbsp low-sodium soy sauce
1 tsp sugar
2 tbsp chopped parsley
½ cup bean sprouts
pinch of salt, optional

Garnish:

shallots,
chopped radish slices

1. Combine all ingredients.

2. Chill.

3. Serve garnished with chopped shallots and radish slices.

Nutritional data per serving:
215 Calories, Carbohydrates 35g, Protein 7g, Fat 5g.

Exchanges per serving: 2 Starch, 1 Vegetable, 1 Fat.

Preparation time: 30 minutes.

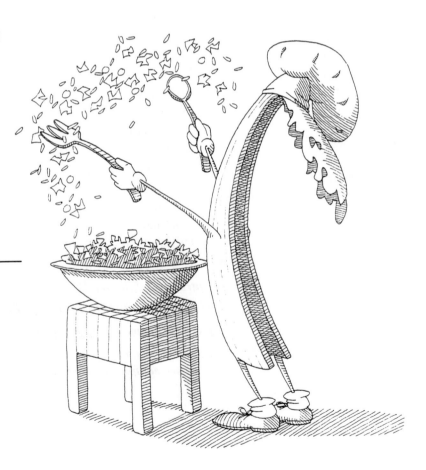

Sauces, Dressings, and Marinades

SAUCES

White Sauce

Serves: 2 cups

2 cups skim milk
1 onion, cut in half
1 small carrot, roughly chopped
1 stalk celery, roughly chopped
1 bay leaf
6 peppercorns
2 tbsp cornstarch

1. Pour milk into saucepan. Add chopped vegetables, bay leaf, and peppercorns.
2. Bring mixture to boil. Immediately reduce heat and simmer for 15 minutes.
3. Strain milk into a bowl. Discard vegetables, bay leaf, and peppercorns.
4. In a separate bowl, mix cornstarch with 2 or 3 tbsp of the warm milk. Stir to make a smooth paste.
5. Gradually add remaining milk to the paste, stirring constantly.
6. Return sauce to the saucepan. Bring to boil, stirring constantly. Reduce heat and simmer gently for 2 minutes, stirring until sauce thickens.
7. Use as required in recipes.

Nutritional data per $1/4$ cup serving:
31 Calories, Carbohydrates 5g, Protein $2^{1}/_{2}$g, Fat .1g.

Exchanges per serving: $1/4$ Skim Milk, $1/8$ Starch.

Preparation time: 20 minutes.
Cooking equipment: medium saucepan.

Cherry Sauce

Makes: 2 cups

2 cups fresh ripe
  cherries, pitted
½ cup Chicken Stock
  (page 80) or ½ cup
  water and 1 stock cube
1 tsp Worcestershire
  sauce
1 tbsp brandy

1. Place 1 cup of cherries into a saucepan or in a microwave bowl with stock and Worcestershire sauce.

2. Boil for 8 minutes until cherries are soft, or microwave on high for 4 minutes. Purée and return to saucepan or bowl.

3. Add remaining cup of cherries and brandy. Simmer for 2 minutes or microwave on high for 2 minutes, and serve.

Nutritional data per ¼ cup serving:
24 Calories, Carbohydrates 6g, Protein 2g, Fat 0g.

Exchanges per serving: ½ Fruit.

Preparation time: 15 minutes.
Cooking equipment: saucepan.

Saté (Peanut) Sauce

Makes: 2 cups

1 tbsp water
1 small onion, grated
1 clove garlic, crushed
½–1 tsp ground chili
¾ cup crunchy peanut
  butter (preferably
  low-salt)
1 tbsp low-sodium soy
  sauce
1 tbsp lemon juice
1¼ cups water

1. In a frying pan, bring water to a boil. Add onion and garlic, and cook gently until soft.

2. Add chili, stir in and cook for 1 minute over medium heat.

3. Add peanut butter and stir well. Add soy sauce, lemon juice, and water, and mix well. Bring mixture to boil, stirring constantly. Reduce heat and simmer gently for 1 minute.

Nutritional data per ¼ cup serving:
46 Calories, Carbohydrates 1g, Protein 1.7g, Fat 4g.

Exchanges per serving: 1 Fat.

Preparation time: 20 minutes.
Cooking equipment: frying pan.

Green Champagne Sauce

Makes: 1 cup

3 kiwi, peeled and
  puréed
½ cup halved green grapes
½ cup champagne

Simple, sophisticated and superb, especially with fish.

1. Place kiwi in saucepan. Add grapes and champagne.
2. Heat gently, but do not boil. Serve immediately.

Nutritional data per ¼ cup serving:
72 Calories, Carbohydrates 11.5g, Protein 1.2g, Fat 0.25g.

Exchanges per serving: ¾ Fruit.

Preparation time: 10 minutes.
Equipment: small-medium saucepan.

Tomato and Basil Sauce

Serves: 4

2 tsp olive oil
1 medium onion, finely
  chopped
1 clove garlic, crushed
1 lb ripe tomatoes, peeled,
  seeded, and chopped
1 tbsp chopped fresh
  basil
½ tsp chopped fresh
  oregano
ground black pepper

1. Heat oil in saucepan, add onion and sauté until translucent.
2. Add garlic and cook for a further 2 minutes.
3. Add tomatoes, herbs and pepper and boil for 8-10 minutes.

Microwave method: Sauté onion until soft (approximately 30 seconds). Add garlic and cook on high for a further 1 minute. Add the tomatoes, herbs, and pepper, and cook on high for 4-6 minutes. Cooking time: 6-8 minutes.

Nutritional data per ¼ cup serving:
48 Calories, Carbohydrates 5g, Protein 1.5g, Fat 2.5g.

Exchanges per serving: ½ Fat, 1 Vegetable.

Preparation time: 20 minutes.
Cooking equipment: medium saucepan.

Cheese Sauce

Makes: 2 cups

8 oz cottage or ricotta
  cheese
½ cup grated low-fat
  Cheddar cheese
½ cup skim milk
1 tbsp cornstarch
1 tbsp skim milk, extra

This versatile and popular sauce works well with any number of savory dishes. It is especially delicious with fish, vegetables or pasta. If you'd like a little more "bite" to the sauce, add ½ tsp prepared English mustard and a pinch of cayenne pepper.

1. Using a food processor or electric blender, blend ricotta or cottage cheese and skim milk until smooth. Add the grated cheese.

2. In saucepan, gently warm the cheese mixture, stirring constantly, until the grated cheese melts.

3. In a cup, blend the cornstarch with the extra tablespoon of milk to make a smooth paste. Add to saucepan and stir into sauce.

4. Stirring constantly, bring sauce to a boil. Immediately reduce heat and simmer gently for 2 minutes, stirring constantly.

Nutritional data per ¼ cup serving:
62 Calories, Carbohydrates 2.6g, Protein 8.5g, Fat 2.3g.

Exchanges per serving: 1¼ Lean Meat.

Preparation time: 10 minutes.
Cooking equipment: medium saucepan, food processor or blender.

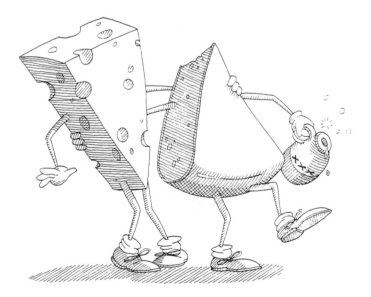

Fresh Vegetable Sauce

Makes: 4 cups

1 apple, peeled and
  grated
1 medium zucchini,
  grated
$\frac{1}{4}$ medium green
  bell pepper,
  finely chopped
1 small onion, finely
  chopped
2 medium tomatoes,
  finely chopped
3 medium mushrooms,
  finely chopped
1 medium carrot, grated
1 clove garlic, crushed
1 tbsp finely chopped
  parsley
$\frac{1}{2}$ tsp finely chopped
  fresh sage or $\frac{1}{4}$ tsp
  dried
$\frac{1}{2}$ tsp finely chopped
  fresh marjoram or $\frac{1}{4}$
  tsp dried
ground black pepper
2 tbsp tomato paste
$\frac{1}{2}$ cup water

Place all ingredients in saucepan, bring to a boil and simmer for 20 minutes. Alternatively, place the ingredients in a microwave-proof bowl, and microwave on high for 10 minutes.

Nutritional data per $\frac{1}{4}$ cup serving:
14 Calories, Carbohydrates 2.5g, Protein 0.8g, Fat 0.1g.

Exchanges per serving: $\frac{1}{2}$ Vegetable.

Preparation time: 30 minutes.
Cooking equipment: medium saucepan.

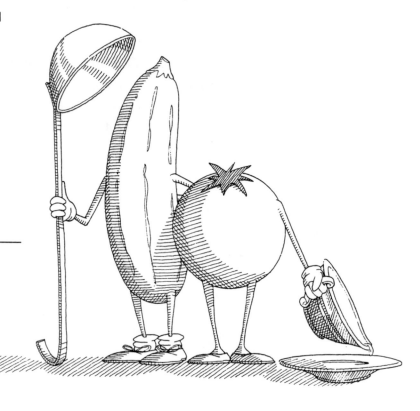

Ratatouille Sauce

Serves: 4

1 small green bell pepper, diced
1 small eggplant peeled, diced
2 small zucchini, diced
2 medium tomatoes, diced, or 16 cherry tomatoes
6 medium mushrooms, diced
1 large onion, peeled and diced
1 clove garlic, crushed
½ tsp dried oregano
black pepper, to taste
3 tbsp water

Ratatouille can be served as a hot vegetable or chilled as a salad. It is also ideal used to surround chicken, veal, or fish fillets during cooking.

Combine all ingredients and cook over low heat for 30 minutes, or microwave on medium for 15 minutes.

Nutritional data per ¼ cup serving:
44 Calories, Carbohydrates 7g, Protein 4g, Fat 1g

Exchanges per serving: 2 Vegetable.

Preparation time: 45 minutes.
Cooking equipment: saucepan.

Black Bean Sauce

Makes: ½ cup

3 tbsp dried black beans
1 clove garlic, crushed
½ tsp finely chopped or minced fresh ginger
1 tbsp brandy or dry sherry
¼ cup water
2 tsp low-sodium soy sauce

Delicious with finely sliced sautéed steak, chicken fillets, or fish.

1. Wash beans thoroughly, drain and mash with garlic, ginger and brandy or sherry.

2. Place in saucepan with water and soy sauce.

3. Bring to a boil, reduce heat and simmer for 2 minutes.

Nutritional data per 2 Tbsp. serving:
45 Calories, Carbohydrates 4g, Protein 4g, Fat 2g.

Exchanges per serving: ⅓ Lean Meat, ¼ Starch.

Preparation time: 7 minutes.
Cooking equipment: small saucepan.

Cucumber and Yogurt Sauce

Makes: 1 cup

½ cucumber, peeled
7 oz low-fat yogurt
1 tsp finely chopped or
   minced fresh ginger
½ tsp minced garlic
1 tbsp lemon juice
¼ tsp freshly ground
   black pepper
¼ tsp mild paprika
1 tbsp chopped parsley
4 cardamom pods,
   crushed

Use this sauce immediately because it will not keep.

1. Grate cucumber, drain well and discard liquid.
2. Combine all the ingredients in a bowl and chill well before serving.

Nutritional data per ¼ cup serving:
30 Calories, Carbohydrates 4g, Protein 2.7g, Fat 0.5g.

Exchanges per serving: ¼ Low-Fat Milk,
⅛ Vegetable.

Preparation time: 15 minutes.

Strawberry and Peppercorn Sauce

Serves: 2 cups

½ cup dry white wine
½ pint strawberries,
   washed, hulled and
   puréed
1 tsp lemon juice
1 tsp brandy
2 tsp green peppercorns
½ cup canned
   evaporated skim milk,
   chilled

Unusual but wonderful with grilled or sautéed chicken fillets, fish, lobster, or crab.

1. Bring wine to the boil and reduce to half by simmering.
2. Add strawberry purée, lemon juice, brandy, and peppercorns.
3. Bring back to boil, simmer 1 minute and set it aside to cool.
4. Whip milk until it is thick. Gradually add the strawberry mixture to it, whipping constantly.
5. Gently reheat the mixture, but do not allow it to boil. Serve immediately.

Nutritional data per ¼ cup serving:
6 Calories, Carbohydrates .9g, Protein .6g, 0 Fat.

Exchanges per serving: ⅛ Milk, ⅛ Fruit.

Preparation time: 15 minutes.
Cooking equipment: medium saucepan.

Sweet and Sour Sauce

Serves: 4

1 large onion
8 shallots
2 medium carrots
1 small red bell pepper, seeded
4 oz mushrooms
2 sticks celery
1 medium cucumber
2 tsp oil
1 clove garlic, crushed
1 tsp grated or minced fresh ginger
2 tbsp tomato paste
$\frac{1}{4}$ cup white vinegar
1 cup water
1 stock cube
$1\frac{1}{2}$ tbsp cornstarch
3 tbsp low-sodium soy sauce
1 tbsp dry sherry
14 oz can of unsweetened pineapple pieces and juice

This is a wonderfully versatile sauce that is just as good served with boiled brown rice or noodles, as it is served with grilled fish, pork, or vegetables.

1. Slice onion, shallots, bell pepper, mushrooms, and celery thinly (about matchstick size).

2. Cut cucumbers into quarters, lengthwise, remove seeds and cut into small pieces of about $\frac{1}{2}$ inch.

3. Heat oil in a large wok or frying pan over high heat. Add garlic and ginger. Stir-fry for 30 seconds, and then add all the other vegetables. Keep heat high and stir-fry for 2-3 minutes until the vegetables are cooked, but still crisp and bright colored.

4. In a bowl, blend tomato paste, vinegar, water, stock cube, cornstarch, soy sauce, and sherry.

5. Drain pineapple pieces, and add the juice to the tomato paste mixture. Keep pineapple aside. Add sauce mixture to the vegetables, and stir until sauce boils and thickens.

6. Add pineapple to the vegetables, and cook for another 3-5 minutes until the pineapple is heated through.

To serve: As an accompaniment serve hot or cold with grilled fish (page 99), or pork and Vegetables en Brochette (page 163). As a light meal serve the sauce with boiled brown rice or noodles.

Nutritional data per serving:
130 Calories, Carbohydrates 22g, Protein 4g, Fat 2.7g.

Exchanges per serving: $2\frac{3}{4}$ Vegetable, $\frac{1}{2}$ Fat, $\frac{1}{2}$ Fruit.

Preparation time: 30 minutes.
Cooking equipment: wok or frying pan.

DRESSINGS

Italian Dressing

Makes: ½ cup

⅓ cup vinegar
1 tbsp lemon juice
1 tbsp chopped parsley
2 tsp chopped chives
1 clove garlic, crushed
½ tsp dry mustard
ground black pepper

Combine ingredients in a screw top jar, shake well and refrigerate.

To store: Cover and refrigerate for up to one week.

Nutritional data per total quantity: negligible.

Preparation time: 5 minutes.

Herbed Tomato Dressing

Makes: 1 cup

½ cup unsweetened
   tomato juice
4 tbsp tomato paste
2 tbsp low-fat yogurt
4 drops Tabasco sauce
1 clove garlic, crushed
1 tbsp chopped parsley
½ tsp chopped fresh
   mixed herbs or ¼ tsp
   mixed dried herbs

Use herbs such as marjoram, basil, or thyme.

1. Combine tomato juice with tomato paste and add to yogurt.

2. Add other ingredients and mix well.

3. Chill and use same day.

Nutritional data per 2 Tbsp. serving:
12 Calories, Carbohydrates 2g, Protein 2g, Fat trace.

Exchanges per serving: ½ Vegetable.

Preparation time: 8 minutes.

Creamy Orange Dressing

Makes: ¾ cup

¼ cup unsweetened
   orange juice
2 tsp orange zest
1 tbsp finely chopped
   parsley
2 tsp finely chopped
   chives
½ cup low-fat yogurt

Combine all ingredients and chill.

Variation: For Creamy Lemon Dressing, prepare as above but omit orange juice and zest, replacing them with 2 tbsp lemon juice.

To store: Cover and refrigerate for up to two days.

Nutritional data per 2 Tbsp. serving:
17 Calories, Carbohydrates 2g, Protein 1.3g, Fat .3g.

Exchanges per serving: ¼ Low-Fat Milk.

Preparation time: 5 minutes.

Curry Dressing

Makes: ½ cup

½ cup low-fat yogurt
2 tsp hot Curry Powder
   or Paste (page 191)
2 tbsp chopped parsley
¼ tsp minced garlic
   (optional)

1. Mix all ingredients and adjust flavorings to taste.

2. Chill and use same day.

Nutritional data per 2 Tbsp. serving:
20 Calories, Carbohydrates 2.2g, Protein 2g, Fat 0.5g.

Exchanges per serving: ⅓ Low-Fat Milk.

Preparation time: 5 minutes.

Orange and Soy Dressing

Makes: ¼ cup

¼ cup unsweetened
   orange juice
2 tsp low-sodium soy sauce
1 clove garlic, crushed
1 tsp oil (optional)

1. Combine all ingredients in a screw top jar.

2. Chill and shake well before use.

To store: Cover and refrigerate for up to two days.

Nutritional data per 2 Tbsp. serving:
32 Calories, Carbohydrates 2g, Protein trace,
Fat 2.5g with oil).

Exchanges per serving: ½ Fat (with oil).

Preparation time: 5 minutes.

Creamy Yogurt Dressing

Makes: ¹/₂ cup

¹/₃ cup low-fat yogurt
2 tbsp lemon juice or
   raspberry vinegar
¹/₂ tsp dry mustard
ground black pepper

Mix all ingredients until smooth. Cover and refrigerate.

To store: Cover and refrigerate for up to three days.

Nutritional data per 2 Tbsp. serving:
11 Calories, Carbohydrates 1.5g, Protein 1g, Fat .25g.

Exchanges per serving: ¹/₈ Milk.

Preparation time: 5 minutes.

Quick and Easy Marinades

Try these marinades with lean beef steaks, lamb cutlets, pork chops or as a marinade for meat on kabobs. Excellent for barbecue or grill. These quantities are for 1 lb of meat and will serve four.

Red Wine Zap:

Combine ¹/₂ cup dry red wine, 1 tbsp tomato paste, 1 tbsp Worcestershire (or soy or teriyaki) sauce, 2 tbsp finely chopped parsley, 1 clove crushed garlic, ground black pepper, to taste, and ¹/₄ tsp finely chopped oregano or basil (optional).

To rev it up—add ¹/₄ cup sweet chili sauce, ¹/₄ cup Worcestershire sauce, or 1-2 cloves crushed garlic. Stir ingredients, and use to brush meat as it grills.

Singapore Sizzler:

Combine 1 tbsp Worcestershire sauce, 1 tbsp soy or teriyaki sauce, 2 tbsp lemon juice, ¹/₄ tsp mustard powder, ¹/₄ tsp ground coriander and ¹/₄ tsp finely chopped green ginger. Stir the ingredients and use to brush meat as it grills.

Spicy Lamb:

Particularly good for lamb is a combination of ¹/₂ cup tomato paste, 2 tsp Worcestershire sauce, 2 tsp chopped fresh or ¹/₂ tsp dried rosemary, dash of Tabasco sauce, and 4 chopped shallots. Stir the ingredients and use to brush meat as it grills.

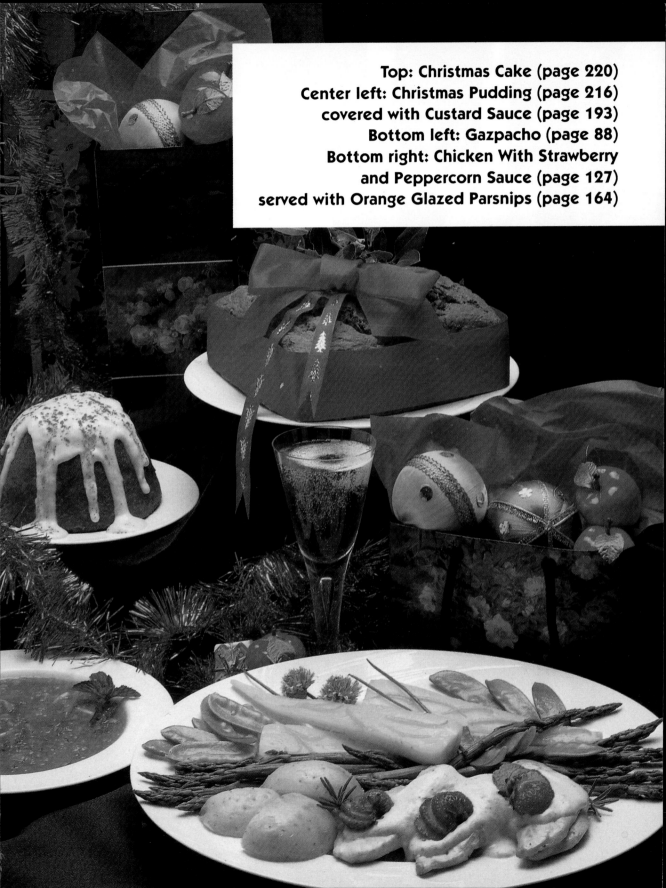

Top: Christmas Cake (page 220)
Center left: Christmas Pudding (page 216)
covered with Custard Sauce (page 193)
Bottom left: Gazpacho (page 88)
Bottom right: Chicken With Strawberry
and Peppercorn Sauce (page 127)
served with Orange Glazed Parsnips (page 164)

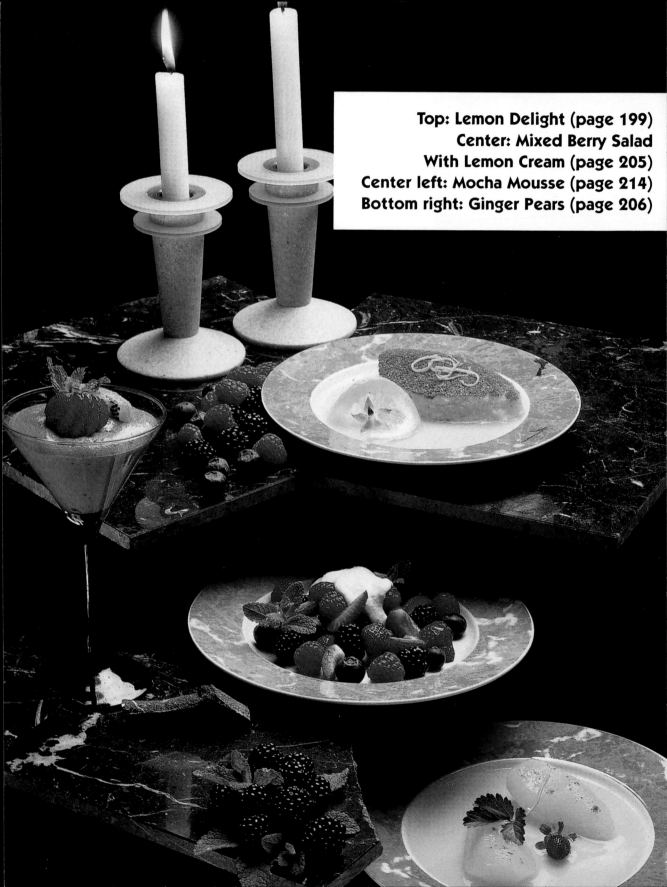

Top: Lemon Delight (page 199)
Center: Mixed Berry Salad
With Lemon Cream (page 205)
Center left: Mocha Mousse (page 214)
Bottom right: Ginger Pears (page 206)

RELISHES AND SEASONINGS

Tomato Relish

Makes: 8 cups

3 large onions
5½ lbs chopped, ripe
  tomatoes
5 granny smith apples,
  cored and chopped
  (skins left on)
3 cups vinegar
1 lb raisins
3 gloves of garlic, crushed
1 cup fresh orange juice
1 tsp mixed spice
1 tsp whole cloves
1 tsp chili powder

1. Place all the ingredients in a large saucepan and bring them to a boil. Turn the heat to low and simmer for 1 hour, stirring frequently. Remove from heat.

2. Pour hot water into clean jars to warm them. Pour water away.

3. Fill jars with hot relish. Allow them to cool, then seal the jars and store.

To store: Keep in sealed jars. Once opened, store in refrigerator.

Nutritional data per 1 cup serving:
263 Calories, Carbohydrates 62.8g, Protein 5.3g, Fat 0.1g.

Exchanges per serving: 1¾ Vegetable, 4 Fruit.

Preparation time: 1½ hours.
Cooking equipment: large saucepan.

Fresh Mango Chutney

Makes: ¾-1 cup

1 ripe medium-large
  mango
2 tsp lemon juice
½ tsp finely chopped or
  minced fresh ginger
1 tbsp raisins

1. Peel mango. Slice flesh from stone and cut into small pieces. Place in a mixing bowl.

2. Add lemon juice, ginger, and raisins.

3. Spoon into glass or plastic container, cover and refrigerate.

To store: Keep in glass or plastic container and refrigerate for up to two days.

Nutritional data per 1 cup serving:
102 Calories, Carbohydrates 24g, Protein 2g, Fat trace.

Exchanges per serving: 1½ Fruit.

Preparation time: 15 minutes.

Plum Sauce

Makes: 8 cups

2 onions, chopped
1 cup water
2 lbs fresh plums, pitted
1 cup fresh orange juice
2 tsp grated or minced
  fresh ginger
6 whole cloves
1 tsp peppercorns
pinch of thyme
pinch of oregano
1 bay leaf

1. Lightly sauté onions in 2-3 tablespoons of the water, for 2 minutes.

2. Add the rest of the ingredients and cook over low heat, stirring regularly.

3. Simmer, with the lid off for at least 1 hour until the mixture thickens.

4. Remove the bay leaf.

5. Pour into clean warmed jars, allow to cool and then seal.

To store: Keep in sealed jars in refrigerator.

Nutritional data per 1 cup serving:
68 Calories, Carbohydrates 15.5g, Protein 1.5g, Fat 0.1g.

Exchanges per serving: 1/4 Vegetable, 1 Fruit.

Preparation time: 1 1/2 hours.
Cooking equipment: large saucepan.

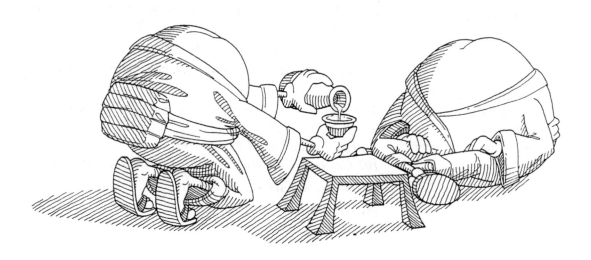

Curry Paste

Makes: ¾ cup

1 tbsp freshly minced or
  grated ginger
2 tbsp ground coriander
1 tbsp ground cinnamon
2 tsp chili powder
1 tbsp powdered
  turmeric
1 tsp minced garlic
1 tbsp lemon juice
2 tbsp vinegar
2 tbsp oil
1 tbsp mustard

You can vary the quantities and ingredients according to taste.

1. Combine ingredients in saucepan and mix to make a smooth paste.

2. Stirring constantly, cook over low heat for 3-4 minutes until slightly thickened.

3. Spoon mixture into a warmed glass jar, seal and store in refrigerator.

To store: Keep in airtight container in refrigerator for up to one month.

Nutritional data per total quantity: negligible.

Preparation time: 6 minutes.
Cooking equipment: saucepan.

Curry Powder

Makes: ¾ cup

½ tsp cayenne pepper
2 tbsp ground coriander
1 tbsp ground cumin
1 tbsp coarsely ground
  black pepper
2 tbsp ground ginger
1 tbsp ground cinnamon
½ tsp ground cloves
¼ tsp ground nutmeg
2 tsp chili powder
2 tbsp powdered
  turmeric

You can vary the ingredients and quantities according to taste. Curry Powder can be stored for a long time, but gradually loses its flavor.

1. Mix ingredients well.

2. Refrigerate in airtight container.

Nutritional data per total quantity: negligible.

Preparation time: 15 minutes.

SWEET SAUCES

Creamy Whipped Topping

Makes: 2 cups

½ cup skim milk powder
1 cup ice water
½ tsp vanilla

Mixture will lose its thickness after 2-3 hours, just re-whip it.

1. Combine all ingredients in a bowl.
2. With electric beater, hand beater or whisk, beat mixture until thick and creamy. Chill.

Nutritional data per total quantity:
163 Calories, Carbohydrates 24g, Protein 16g, Fat 1g.

Exchanges per total quantity: 2 Skim Milk.

Preparation time: 10 minutes.

Blueberry Sauce

Serves: 4

1 cup blueberries, fresh
  or frozen
½ cup orange juice
½ tsp cinammon
1 tbsp brown sugar
2 tsp cornstarch
1 tbsp water

1. Place berries, juice, cinammon, and sugar into a saucepan. Bring to a boil, then remove from heat.
2. Combine cornstarch and water, making sure there are no lumps.
3. Stir into the berries, then reheat until the mixture thickens.
4. Spoon hot sauce over pancakes.

Nutritional data per serving:
52 Calories, Carbohydrates 13g, Protein 0.4g, Fat trace.

Exchanges per serving: 1 Fruit.

Peparation time: 15 minutes.
Cooking equipment: saucepan.

Custard Sauce

Serves: 4

3 level tbsp cornstarch
1 egg, beaten
18 fl oz skim milk
2 tsp vanilla extract
2 tsp sugar, Equal or
  other artificial sweetener

You can serve this sauce hot or cold.

1. Blend cornstarch, beaten egg, and a small quantity of the milk to make a smooth paste.
2. Place remaining milk in saucepan and bring to boil.
3. Gradually stir in cornstarch paste. Continue stirring until mixture thickens.
4. Simmer for 1 minute, stirring constantly.
5. Add vanilla and sugar, Equal or other artificial sweetener.

Nutritional data per serving:
71 Calories, Carbohydrates 13g, Protein 5g, Fat trace.

Exchanges per serving: ½ Skim Milk, ¼ Starch.

Preparation time: 15 minutes.
Cooking equipment: saucepan.

Variation:

Orange Custard Sauce

Follow the recipe for custard sauce and add 1 tsp of finely grated orange rind to milk before heating.

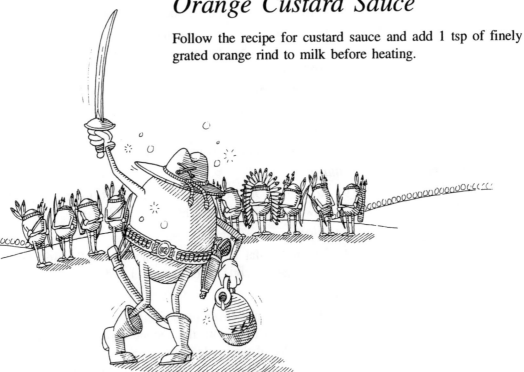

Desserts

Apple Layer Cake

Serves: 10-12

Cake:

1 cup whole wheat
pastry flour
1½ tsp baking powder
½ tsp salt (optional)
4 oz low-fat cream cheese
1 egg
1 tsp vanilla extract
2 tsp brown sugar

Filling:

2½ cups cold, stewed
apple, flavored with
lemon zest, cinnamon,
and cloves to taste

Topping:

4 oz low-fat cream cheese
2 tsp sugar
zest of ½ lemon
4 oz ricotta cheese
¼ tsp ground cinnamon

Decoration:

2 oz chopped pecans

Refrigerate this glorious cake for a day before you serve it so that it is easy to cut and the filling has developed its full flavor.

Cake:

1. Sift flour into bowl. Return bran to sifted flour. Add baking powder and salt.

2. Soften cheese, and beat with a spoon until smooth. Add egg and vanilla and beat again. Add sugar and mix well.

3. Gradually blend flour into cheese mixture until a soft dough is formed.

4. Turn out onto a floured board and knead into a ball.

5. Divide into three. Shape and roll into rounds approximately 10 inches in diameter, making them as equal as possible.

6. Lift onto very lightly greased baking sheets.

7. Bake for 12 minutes until cooked through and light brown.

8. Remove and cool on cake racks.

Filling:

9. Add lemon zest, cinnamon, and cloves (to taste) to cold, stewed apple. Mixture should be fairly firm.

Topping:

10. Soften low-fat cream cheese until smooth. Add sugar, lemon zest, ricotta, and cinnamon and mix well.

Assembly:

11. Place one cake layer on serving plate. Cover with half the apple. Cover with the second layer, spread with the remainder of the apple, then place third layer on top.

12. Spread topping mixture on top and sides of cake.

13. Sprinkle with pecans, cover with plastic film and refrigerate for at least 24 hours.

14. Cut into wedges to serve.

Nutritional data per serving (if 10 servings):
182 Calories, Carbohydrates 17g, Protein 6g, Fat 10g.

Exchanges per serving: 1 Medium-Fat Meat, 1 Starch,
¼ Fruit, ½ Fat.

Preparation time: cake 30 minutes, assembly 30 minutes, begin preparation 24 hours before serving.
Cooking equipment: 2 baking sheets.
Oven temperature: 350°F.

Old-Fashioned Dumplings

Serves: 4

¾ cup skim or low-fat milk
¼ tsp ground nutmeg
½ cup semolina
1 egg
1 tsp vanilla extract
1 tbsp sugared zest (lemon, lime, or orange)
1 tbsp currants
1 tbsp raisins
small quantity of unbleached flour
1 cup Orange Custard Sauce (page 193) or 1 cup apple purée

1. Place milk and nutmeg in small saucepan and bring to boil.

2. Remove from heat and quickly stir in semolina.

3. Return to heat and stir for one minute.

4. Add egg, vanilla, peel, currants, and raisins and mix well.

5. Turn onto a lightly floured board and knead gently until smooth.

6. Break off small, even-sized pieces and roll into balls the size of large marbles. Toss each ball in flour.

7. Half fill a large saucepan with water and bring to boil.

8. Drop dumplings into boiling water and cook for approximately 5 minutes. (Note: the dumplings will rise to the top of the water as they cook.)

9. Drain and serve immediately with Orange Custard Sauce or apple purée.

Nutritional data per serving:
140 Calories, Carbohydrates 24g, Protein 7g, Fat 2g.

Exchanges per serving: 1 Starch, ½ Fruit, ¼ Milk.

Preparation time: 20 minutes plus preparation time for sauce.
Cooking equipment: small saucepan, large saucepan.

Fruit Strudel

Serves: 4

6 sheets filo pastry
2 tbsp skim milk
4 apples, peeled and
    very finely sliced
4 tbsp raisins
2 tbsp chopped pecan
    nuts
1 tsp cinnamon
¼ tsp ground cloves
1 tbsp brown sugar

All the pleasure of the traditional strudel, but with a fraction of the fat.

1. Spread out 2 sheets of pastry. Brush lightly with milk.
2. Place another 2 layers of pastry on top. Again brush with milk.
3. Repeat for remaining two sheets of pastry.
4. Sprinkle remaining ingredients over the pastry.
5. Spray a baking tray with non-stick baking spray. Carefully roll up the pastry. Place on the baking tray, loose edge down.
6. Brush the strudel well with milk. Bake for 25-30 minutes.

Serve warm, cut in thick slices. You may serve this with Creamy Whipped Topping (page 192).

Nutritional data per serving:
191 Calories, Carbohydrates 36g, Protein 5g, Fat 5g.

Exchanges per serving: 1 Starch, 1¼ Fruit, 1 Fat.

Preparation time: 45 minutes.
Cooking equipment: baking tray.
Oven temperature: 400°F.

Banana Strudel

The basic method is exactly the same as for Fruit Strudel (see above); only the filling is different. For this delectable filling combine:

4 ripe bananas (sliced), 4 tbsp raisins, 1 tsp cinnamon, 4 tbsp shredded coconut, 2 tbsp unsweetened orange juice, 2 tbsp chopped pecan nuts or walnuts, 4 tbsp brown rum and 1 tsp brown sugar.

Nutritional data per serving:
263 Calories, Carbohydrates 43g, Protein 7g, Fat 9g.

Exchanges per serving: 1½ Fruit, 1½ Fat, 1 Starch.

Apricot Strudel

The basic method is exactly the same as for Fruit Strudel (see page 196); only the filling is different. Here you combine: 1 lb apricots (pitted and sliced) or 1 can (15 oz) of unsweetened apricot pieces, 4 tbsp raisins, 2 tbsp slivered almonds, 1 tsp cinnamon and 1 tbsp brown sugar.

Nutritional data per serving:
138 Calories, Carbohydrates 22g, Protein 5g, Fat 5g.

Exchanges per serving: 1 Starch, ½ Fruit, 1 Fat.

Ricotta Raisin Flan

Serves: 6-8

2 tbsp margarine
4 oz shredded whole wheat crackers, crushed
1 lb ricotta cheese
4 tbsp apple concentrate
1 cup raisins, chopped
zest of 1 lemon
½ tsp ground cinnamon
¼ tsp ground nutmeg
1 egg
½ cup low-fat milk
Garnish: ground cinnamon

1. Melt margarine, then add cracker crumbs and mix.
2. Spread over base and up sides of pie dish. Press well to make an even, firm crust.
3. Bake 10 minutes. Cool.
4. Mix ricotta, apple concentrate, raisins, lemon zest, and spices.
5. Beat egg and combine with milk. Mix it with other ingredients. Blend well.
6. Pour into pie dish. Bake for 30-45 minutes until set and lightly browned.
7. Sprinkle with a little cinnamon and serve.

To store: Cover and refrigerate for up to two days.

Nutritional data per serving:
373 Calories, Carbohydrates 43 g, Protein 13 g, Fat 17 g.

Exchanges per serving: 1½ Medium-Fat Meat, 1 Fat (poly), 1 Starch, 2 Fruit.

Preparation time: 1 hour 50 minutes.
Cooking equipment: small saucepan, pie dish.
Oven temperature: 350°F.

Lemon and Cinnamon Cheesecake

Serves: 8

Crust:

1 cup shredded
  whole wheat cracker
  crumbs
2 oz almonds, crushed
1 tbsp margarine, melted
2 tsp water
2 tsp cinnamon

Filling:

10 fl oz buttermilk
8 oz ricotta cheese
juice of 2 lemons
zest of 1 lemon
1 tsp vanilla extract
1 tbsp sugar or Equal
  or other equivalent
  artificial sweetener
1 tbsp powdered gelatin
2 tbsp water

Garnish:

kiwi
strawberries (optional)
2 tsp cinnamon

You must make this recipe the day before you want to serve it to allow the filling to set.

Crust:

1. Combine all ingredients for biscuit base.

2. Press mixture into a lined pie dish and refrigerate for 30 minutes.

Filling:

3. Mix buttermilk with ricotta cheese, lemon juice, lemon zest, vanilla extract, and sugar or artificial sweetener. Beat until smooth and fluffy.

4. Dissolve gelatin in hot water. Cool slightly and fold into buttermilk mixture and blend well.

5. Pour into pie base and refrigerate until set.

6. Next day, decorate with sliced kiwi and a sprinkle of cinnamon.

Variation: Replace lemons and lemon zest with the juice and zest of 1 orange.

To store: Cover and refrigerate for up to three days.

Nutritional data per serving:
191 Calories, Carbohydrates 14g, Protein 7g, Fat 12g.

Exchanges per serving: 1 Medium-Fat Meat, 1 Starch, 1 Fat.

Preparation time: 1 hour, including chilling time for the base. Cooking equipment: pie dish with removable base, electric beater.

Lemon Delight

3 eggs
5 tbsp fresh lemon juice
zest of 1 lemon
1 tbsp melted butter
3 tbsp whole wheat
  unbleached flour
1½ cups low-fat milk
1 tbsp sugar or Equal

Preparation time: 1 hour.
Cooking equipment:
  individual baking dishes,
  large baking dish for
  water bath.
Oven temperature: 325°F.

1. Separate eggs. Beat egg whites until stiff peaks form.
2. Beat yolks with the remaining ingredients until smooth.
3. Gradually fold the egg whites into mixture.
4. Spoon evenly into four baking dishes.
5. Place in a larger baking dish. Carefully pour water into the larger baking dish until it reaches two-thirds up the outside of the individual baking dishes.
6. Bake for approximately 20 minutes or until set and lightly browned.
7. Cool slightly in the water-filled dish to prevent shrinking.

To store: Cover and refrigerate for 1 day only.

Nutritional data per serving:
212 Calories, Carbohydrates 12g, Protein 9g, Fat 14g.

Exchanges per serving: ¾ *Medium-Fat Meat, 1 Fat,*
¼ *Starch,* ½ *Low-Fat Milk.*

Fruity Baked Rice Pudding

3½ cups skim milk
5 tbsp uncooked brown
  or white rice
1 tbsp sugar
4 tbsp raisins
4 tbsp dried peaches or
  apricots
Garnish: ground nutmeg
  or cinnamon

1. Combine milk, rice and sugar, and place mixture in baking dish. Cover and bake for 45 minutes.
2. Remove from oven, add dried fruit and stir.
3. Leave uncovered and return to oven. Cook for another 45-60 minutes until rice is cooked. A skin will form on top of rice.
4. Serve hot or cold, garnished with ground nutmeg or cinnamon.

To store: Cover and refrigerate for up to three days.

Nutritional data per serving:
191 Calories, Carbohydrates 38g, Protein 9g, Fat trace.

Exchanges per serving: ¾ *Milk, 1 Fruit,* ¾ *Starch.*

Preparation time: 2 hours.
Cooking equipment: baking dish with lid.
Oven temperature: 350°F.

Spiced Oranges

Serves: 4

1 cup red wine, such as claret or burgundy
½ cup unsweetened orange juice
¼ tsp ground cinnamon or 1 cinnamon stick
3 oranges
Equal or other artificial sweetener to taste

The ideal dessert after a long hot summer's day.

1. Place wine, orange juice, and cinnamon in a saucepan and bring to a boil.
2. Boil hard for 2 minutes, then remove from heat, or microwave on high for 2-3 minutes.
3. Peel and thinly slice oranges, removing all pith and seeds, and arrange in a glass serving bowl.
4. Pour wine mixture over oranges, discarding cinnamon stick.
5. Chill well and sweeten before serving.

To store: Cover and refrigerate for up to four days.

Nutritional data per serving:
52 Calories, Carbohydrates 11g, Protein 1g, Fat trace.

Exchanges per serving: 1 Fruit.

Preparation time: 15 minutes.
Cooking equipment: saucepan.

Creamy Rice

Serves: 4

1 cup uncooked basmati rice
1½ cups water
2½ cups skim or low-fat milk
½ cup raisins
½ tsp ground nutmeg
1 tsp vanilla extract
2 packets of Equal or artificial sweetener equivalent to 4 tsp of sugar

1. Wash rice and place in saucepan. Cover with the water, and simmer over very low heat until water is absorbed.
2. Add 1 cup milk. Simmer again until absorbed.
3. Add the remaining 1½ cups milk and cook again until the milk is absorbed.
4. Stir in raisins, nutmeg, vanilla, and sweetener (to taste).
5. Serve warm with sliced stewed or fresh fruit.

To store: Cover and refrigerate for up to three days.

Nutritional data per serving:
283 Calories, Carbohydrates 58g, Protein 10g, Fat 1g.

Exchanges per serving: 2½ Starch, ½ Skim Milk, 1 Fruit.

Preparation time: 1 hour.
Cooking equipment: saucepan.

Sweet Potato and Pecan Pie

Serves: 8

15 shredded whole wheat
   crackers, crushed
3 tbsp margarine, melted
2 cups mashed cooked
   sweet potato
4 tbsp lemon juice
1 tsp cinnamon
½ tsp nutmeg
¼ tsp ground ginger
¼ tsp ground cloves
3 tbsp brown sugar
pinch salt
1 cup low-fat milk
4 oz pecans, chopped
2 eggs, separated

1. Line a pie or flan dish with aluminum foil.

2. Mix crushed crackers with margarine and spoon into dish. Spread over base and up the sides, pressing with the back of a spoon.

3. Bake for 10-15 minutes, then remove and cool.

4. Spoon sweet potato into a mixing bowl. Add lemon juice, spices, ginger, sugar, and salt and stir well to combine.

5. Stir in milk, chopped pecan, and egg yolks.

6. Beat egg whites until soft peaks form, then fold into sweet potato mixture.

7. Spoon into crumb crust and bake for 45-60 minutes, or until set and lightly browned. Serve warm or cold.

Nutritional data per portion:
344 Calories, Carbohydrates 31g, Protein 7g, Fat 22g.

Exchanges per serving: 2 Starch, 4 Fat.

Preparation time: 1½ hours.
Cooking equipment: saucepan, pie dish.
Oven temperature: 350°F.

Baked Custard

Serves: 4

2 eggs
liquid artificial sweetener
   to taste
1⅓ cups skim milk
1 tsp vanilla extract
sprinkling of ground
   nutmeg

This family favorite can be served hot or cold.

1. In bowl, lightly beat the eggs.

2. Gradually add the milk to the egg mixture, stirring constantly. Stir in the vanilla extract and sweetener.

3. Pour mixture into a pie or soufflé dish or dishes. Sprinkle with nutmeg.

4. Stand the baking dish(es) in a large baking dish. Carefully pour enough water into the large baking dish to reach two-thirds up the outside of the pie or soufflé dish(es).

5. Bake for 35 minutes if you are using individual dishes, 45 minutes if you are using one big dish. The custard should be lightly browned and set in the center.

Nutritional data per serving:
63 Calories, Carbohydrates 4g, Protein 6g, Fat 3g.

Exchanges per serving: ½ Medium-Fat Meat, ⅓ Skim Milk.

Preparation time: 1 hour 10 minutes.
Cooking equipment: deep pie or soufflé dish or four single-serve oven-proof dishes, large baking dish for water bath.
Oven temperature: 300°F.

Fruit Crumble

Serves: 4

3 large cooking apples, peeled cored and sliced
2 tbsp water
½ tsp ground cinnamon or 3 cloves
Topping:
1⅓ cups Meg's Muesli (page 66)
or
½ cup rolled oats
2 tbsp shredded coconut
2 tbsp mixed dried fruit
2 tsp chopped nuts
¼ cup bran flakes
¼ cup All-Bran

You can replace the apples in this recipe with peaches, apricots, or plums or with two apples and half a cup of cooked rhubarb. If you have a favorite combination, you can use it in this recipe, too.

1. Place apple into a saucepan, add water, and cinnamon or cloves.
2. Gently simmer for approximately 10 minutes until apple is tender, or microwave, covered, on high for 6 minutes.
3. Lightly grease a small casserole and spoon in apple, removing cloves if used.
4. Mix topping ingredients and sprinkle thickly over apple.
5. Bake for 30 minutes or until topping becomes golden.
6. Serve hot or cold.

To store: Cover and refrigerate for up to 4 days.

Nutritional data per serving:
245 Calories, Carbohydrates 38g, Protein 7g, Fat 7g.

Exchanges per serving: 1 Fruit, 1½ Starch, 1 Fat.

Preparation time: 1 hour.
Cooking equipment: saucepan, small casserole.
Oven temperature: 350°F.

Summer Pudding

Serves: 4

14 slices whole wheat bread
6 cups mixed fresh berries (strawberries, raspberries, blueberries, loganberries)
4 tsp sugar
Garnish: extra berries

1. Cut crusts off bread and discard them.
2. Cut 4 round bases and tops out of crustless bread. Set tops aside. Place a base in each individual soufflé dish. Use the remaining bread to line the sides of the dishes. Do this carefully, making sure that there are no gaps.
3. Wash and hull berries. Chop strawberries.
4. Place berries and sugar in saucepan, and heat gently until liquid runs from berries.
5. Fill soufflé dishes, packing fruit down firmly, and pour juice over.
6. Cover each with one of the reserved tops.
7. Place a weight on top and refrigerate overnight.
8. Remove and discard the tops.
9. Turn onto serving dishes. Garnish with extra berries.

Nutritional data per serving:
209 Calories, Carbohydrates 42g, Protein 7g, Fat 1g.

Exchanges per serving: 2 Starch, 1 Fruit.

Preparation time: 20 minutes, plus overnight standing time.
Cooking equipment: 4 individual soufflé dishes, saucepan.

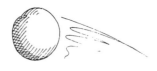

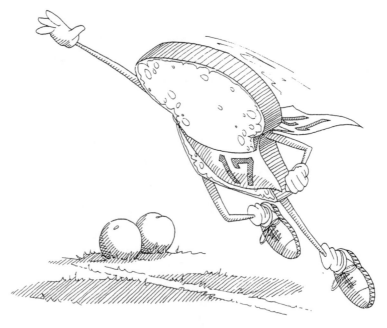

Pumpkin Pie

Serves: 6

Pastry:
2 tbsp margarine
1 cup whole wheat flour
1 egg yolk
juice of ½ lemon plus
  cold water to make
  ⅓ cup

Filling:
2 cups firm pumpkin
  purée
¼ cup ricotta cheese
¼ cup low-fat yogurt
½ cup skim or low-fat
  milk
2 eggs, separated
½ tsp nutmeg
1 tsp cinnamon
¼ tsp ginger
¼ tsp ground cloves
juice and zest of 1 lemon
Equal or other artificial
  sweetener to taste
Garnish: ground
  cinnamon

Pastry:

1. Rub margarine into flour until mixture resembles fine bread-crumbs.

2. Mix egg yolk with juice and water.

3. Mix liquid into flour with a knife, to make a soft dough.

4. Turn out onto floured board. Knead lightly, leave for 15 minutes.

5. Roll out on floured board, then cover base and sides of pie dish with pastry. Add a second strip around top edge and pinch as a decorative edge. Prick pastry and place in oven, bake for approximately 1 hour until lightly browned. Remove and cool.

Filling:

6. Combine in a bowl pumpkin, ricotta, yogurt, milk, and egg yolks. Beat well.

7. Add spices, lemon juice and zest, and sweetener. Check taste and adjust if necessary.

8. Beat egg whites until soft peaks form, fold into pumpkin mixture.

9. Pour into pastry shell and bake in a preheated oven until set (about 1 hour).

10. Sprinkle with a little cinnamon to serve.

Variation: Fold ¼ cup chopped pecans into filling.

To store: Cover and refrigerate for up to two days.

Nutritional data per serving:
203 Calories, Carbohydrates 20g, Protein 9g, Fat 10g.

Exchanges per serving: ¾ Medium-Fat Meat, 1 Fat, 1 Starch, ⅓ Fruit.

Preparation time: 2 hours. Cooking equipment: pie dish. Oven temperature: 350°F.

Mixed Berry Salad with Lemon Cream

Serves: 4

Salad:

1 cup strawberries
1 cup blackberries
1 cup blueberries
¼ cup unsweetened
  apple juice

Lemon cream:

8 oz ricotta cheese
3 oz low-fat yogurt
zest of 1 lemon
2 tsp brown sugar

When berries are in season, celebrate with this salad dressed with smooth lemon cream.

1. Wash and hull berries, slice strawberries if large.
2. Place in bowl and pour apple juice over.
3. Chill in refrigerator.

Lemon cream:

4. Mix ricotta, yogurt, lemon zest, and sugar.
5. Chill.
6. Spoon lemon cream over fruit and serve.

Variation: Replace blackberries with loganberries.

Nutritional data per serving:
100 Calories, Carbohydrates 20g, Protein 4g, Fat 1g.

Exchanges per serving: 1 Medium-Fat Meat, 1 Fruit.

Preparation time: 30 minutes.

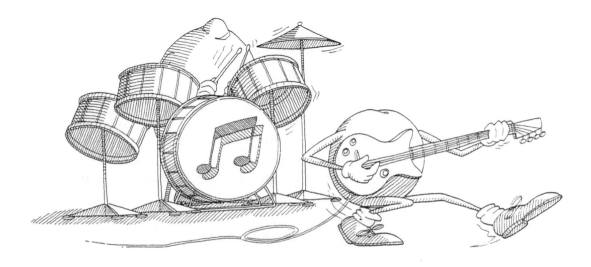

Hot Jamaican Pineapple

Serves: 4

½ medium pineapple, cut lengthwise with top intact
3 bananas, peeled and chopped
4 tsp brown rum
2 tsp brown sugar
¼ cup shredded coconut

1. Cut pineapple out of skin, being careful not to pierce skin. Scoop out any remaining pulp and juice and retain.

2. Chop pineapple into chunks, discarding core. Add to pulp and juice in bowl. Add bananas. Add rum and brown sugar.

3. Spoon fruit and juices into shell and sprinkle with coconut.

4. Place in baking dish, and bake for 30-45 minutes until fruit is heated through and coconut is toasted.

5. Spoon into serving dishes.

Nutritional data per serving:
130 Calories, Carbohydrates 25g, Protein 2g, Fat 2g.

Exchanges per serving: 1½ Fruit, ½ Fat.

Preparation time: 1 hour.
Cooking equipment: baking dish.
Oven temperature: 350°C.

Ginger Pears

Serves: 4

4 medium pears, peeled and quartered
10 fl oz low-calorie dry ginger ale
juice of 1 lemon
½ tsp minced fresh ginger
¼ cup orange juice concentrate
3–4 drops yellow food coloring (optional)
6 cloves
ground cinnamon

1. Place pears in saucepan. Add ginger ale, lemon juice, ginger, orange juice concentrate, food coloring, and cloves.

2. Cover and simmer until pears are tender, turning and basting the pears so they cook and color evenly. Alternatively microwave, covered, on high for 4-6 minutes until tender.

3. Lift pears onto serving dish.

4. Simmer juice until slightly reduced.

5. Pour over pears. Sprinkle with cinnamon.

6. Serve hot or chilled.

To store: Cover and refrigerate for up to four days.

Nutritional data per serving:
91 Calories, Carbohydrates 22g, Protein 1g, Fat 0g.

Exchanges per serving: 1½ Fruit.

Preparation time: 1 hour.
Cooking equipment: saucepan.

Baked Apples with Orange and Strawberry Sauce

Serves: 4

4 granny smith apples
cinnamon
1 cup orange juice
1 pint strawberries
liquid artificial
  sweetener to taste
Garnish:
2 tbsp slivered almonds
  or chopped pecans
orange slices

1. Peel and core apples. When peeling leave some peel on to create a horizontal striped effect.

2. Place in a small baking dish. Sprinkle cinnamon over, then orange juice.

3. Bake, covered, for 30-35 minutes, or microwave on high for 6-8 minutes, until tender but still retaining their shape. Baste occasionally to prevent drying out.

4. While apples are cooking, wash and hull strawberries and purée them. Add sweetener to purée.

5. When apples are cooked, lift gently onto individual serving dishes.

6. Reduce cooking liquid by boiling if necessary, and pour into strawberry purée. Mix and pour over apples.

7. Decorate with slivered nuts and orange slices.

8. Serve warm or chilled.

To store: Cover and refrigerate for up to two days.

Nutritional data per serving:
92 Calories, Carbohydrates 18g, Protein 2g, Fat 1g.

Exchanges per serving: $1^1/_2$ **Fruit,** $^1/_2$ **Fat.**

Preparation time: 1 hour.
Cooking equipment: food processor, baking dish, small saucepan.
Oven temperature: 350°F.

English Fruit Compote

Serves: 4

1 small apple, peeled, cored and cut into 8 wedges

1 cup unsweetened canned peaches in natural juice, made up of approximately ½ cup peaches and ½ cup liquid

1 small pear, peeled, cored and cut into 8 wedges

12 whole cherries

4 yellow plums, cut in half and pitted

4 cloves

pinch ground cinnamon

This is usually a chilled dessert, but you can serve it hot. Vary the fruit according to season and your preference. For instance, if fresh plums are not available, use canned, unsweetened apricot halves or peach slices, which you add after the other fruit has been cooked.

1. Place ingredients in saucepan, with apple at the bottom and peaches on the top.
2. Bring to a boil and simmer gently for 10 minutes or until all fruit is tender.
3. Cool and place in refrigerator for at least 2 hours before serving in glass dishes.

Microwave method: Place fruit in microwave dish, cover and cook on medium for 5 minutes.

To store: Cover and refrigerate for up to three days.

Nutritional data per serving:
68 Calories, Carbohydrates 16g, Protein 1g, Fat 0g.

Exchanges per serving: 1 Fruit.

Preparation time: 2 hours 20 minutes, including cooling time.

Cooking equipment: medium saucepan.

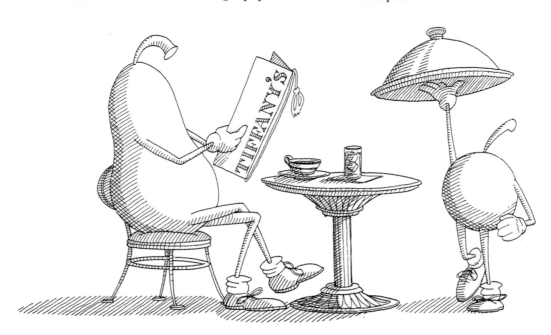

Flambéed Pancakes or Crêpes

Serves: 4

A mixture of fruits (for
instance: 1 pint
strawberries, washed
and hulled; 2 bananas,
sliced; 8 apricots, pitted
and quartered)
juice of 1 orange
½ tsp ground cinnamon
4 tbsp brandy
8 Pancakes (page 95)
   or 12 Crêpes (page 94),
   warmed

1. In a frying pan, combine fruit and juice and simmer gently for approximately 5 minutes until fruit heats through and softens.
2. Drain off juice and set aside.
3. Add brandy to pan, heat and ignite with a match or lighter. Stir fruit gently and allow brandy to burn out.
4. Pour juice back into pan and reheat.
5. Divide fruit evenly between pancakes or crêpes and roll up or, if using crêpes, fold into four to make triangles.

Nutritional data per serving:
296 Calories, Carbohydrates 59g, Protein 12g, Fat 5g.

Exchanges per serving: 2 Starch, 2 Fruit.

Preparation time: 10 minutes.
Cooking equipment: frying pan.

Berry and Cheese Pancakes

Serves: 4

2 cups mixed berries,
   washed and hulled
1 tsp water
8 Pancakes (page 95),
   warmed
8 tbsp cottage cheese

1. Poach berries in water for approximately 3 minutes until soft.
2. Divide fruit evenly between pancakes and top each with 1 tbsp cottage cheese.
3. Roll up and serve hot.

Nutritional data per serving:
266 Calories, Carbohydrates 29g, Protein 16g, Fat 9g.

Exchanges per serving: ¾ Lean Meat, 1 Fruit, 1 Starch, 1 Fat.

Preparation time: 5 minutes.
Cooking equipment: frying pan.

Apple and Raisin Pancakes

Serves: 4

4 apples, peeled, cored
   and sliced
2 cloves
2 tbsp raisins
8 Pancakes (page 95),
   warmed

1. Poach apples gently in a little water with cloves and raisins for approximately 5 minutes until soft. Alternatively, microwave, covered, on high for 5-8 minutes.
2. Remove cloves and divide apple mixture evenly between pancakes.
3. Roll up and serve hot.

Nutritional data per serving:
283 Calories, Carbohydrates 50g, Protein 10g, Fat 5g.
Exchanges per serving: 2 Starch, 1 Fruit, 1 Fat.
Preparation time: 10 minutes. Cooking equipment: saucepan.

Buckwheat Pancakes with Blueberry Sauce

Makes 8 pancakes (2 per serving)

½ cup buckwheat flour
½ cup unbleached flour
2 tsp baking powder
½ tsp cinnamon
1 tbsp sugar
1 egg, beaten
¾ cup low-fat milk
2 cups Blueberry
   Sauce (page 192)

1. Sift flours, baking powder, and cinnamon into a mixing bowl. Return any husks to bowl.
2. Add sugar and mix in well.
3. Beat eggs and milk together.
4. Stir egg mixture slowly into the center of the flour mixture, bringing flour in from the sides as you mix, then beat well until there are no lumps.
5. Heat frying pan, spraying with a little baking spray to prevent sticking.
6. Spoon 2 tablespoons of the mixture into pan, cooking 2 pancakes at a time. When bubbles appear on the surface, turn the pancakes and cook on the other side until golden brown.
7. Keep warm until all pancakes are cooked.
8. Serve with Blueberry Sauce spooned over.

Nutritional data per serving (4 servings):
165 Calories, Carbohydrates 28g, Protein 7.5g, Fat 2.5g.
Exchanges per serving: 1 Starch, 1 Fruit, ¼ Low-Fat Milk.
Preparation time: 30 minutes.
Cooking equipment: frying pan.

Crêpes Suzette

Serves: 4

4 oranges, peeled and
   cut into segments, pith
   removed
juice of 1 orange
3 tbsp brandy
12 crêpes (page 94),
   warmed
Garnish: zest of 1 orange

1. Poach orange segments gently in orange juice until heated through.
2. Drain off juice and set aside.
3. Add brandy to fruit in frying pan, heat and ignite with a match or a lighter. Stir fruit gently and allow brandy to burn out.
5. Pour juice back into pan and reheat.
6. Place crêpes one by one in pan, filling each with fruit, and folding each into four to make a triangle. This allows crêpes to absorb the juice.
7. Serve topped with sprinkling of orange zest.

Nutritional data per serving:
237 Calories, Carbohydrates 37g, Protein 10g, Fat 5g.

Exchanges per serving: 1 Fruit, 1½ Starch.

Preparation time: 10 minutes
Cooking equipment: large frying pan.

Queen's Pudding

Serves: 4

4 eggs
1 pint skim or low-fat milk
2 tsp vanilla extract
3 slices whole wheat
   bread, crumbed
4 tbsp strawberry or
   raspberry purée
1 tbsp sugar

If you do not have any strawberry or raspberry purée, you can use low-calorie jam as a substitute.

1. Separate 2 eggs and put egg whites aside.
2. Combine egg yolks with other 2 whole eggs and beat.
3. Add milk and vanilla.
4. Distribute bread crumbs evenly between four individual baking dishes.
5. Pour equal amounts of custard mixture into each dish.
6. Put individual dishes in a larger baking dish, and carefully pour in water until it reaches two-thirds up the outside of the individual baking dishes. Bake for 30-45 minutes.
7. When cooked, carefully spread top of custard with fruit purée.
8. Beat the remaining 2 egg whites until they are stiff and fold in sugar and pile over purée.

9. Bake for about 5 minutes until meringue is lightly browned.

To store: Cover and refrigerate for up to 2 days.

Nutritional data per serving:
189 Calories, Carbohydrates 21g, Protein 13g, Fat 6g.

Exchanges per serving: 1 Medium-Fat Meat, ½ Skim Milk, ¾ Starch, ¼ Fruit.

Preparation time: 1½ hours.
Cooking equipment: individual baking dishes, large baking dish for water bath.
Oven temperature: 350°F.

Golden Fruit Flummery

Serves: 12

1 pkt low-calorie gelatin, orange or orange and mango flavors
1½ cups boiling water
½ cup canned evaporated skim milk, chilled
13 oz can solid packed unsweetened peach pieces, puréed
1 large mango puréed
Garnish: Creamy Whipped Topping (page 192), sprig of mint

To prevent the evaporated milk separating from the rest of the flummery, you need to have the gelatin and milk mixtures at approximately the same temperature before you combine them. Vary this recipe by a puréeing a 13 oz can solid packed unsweetened apricot pieces instead of peaches and mango.

1. Dissolve gelatin in boiling water, cool, place in refrigerator until just beginning to set.

2. Whip jelly and, as it becomes fluffy, slowly add evaporated skim milk, whipping continually until the mixture thickens.

3. Gently mix in puréed fruit and pour into glass dishes.

4. Chill well before serving. Garnish with a spoonful of whipped topping and a sprig of mint on each.

To store: Cover and refrigerate for up to three days.

Nutritional data per serving:
31 Calories, Carbohydrates 6g, Protein 2g, Fat trace.

Exchanges per serving: ½ Fruit.

Preparation time: 2 hours (including time taken to chill jelly).
Cooking equipment: electric beater.

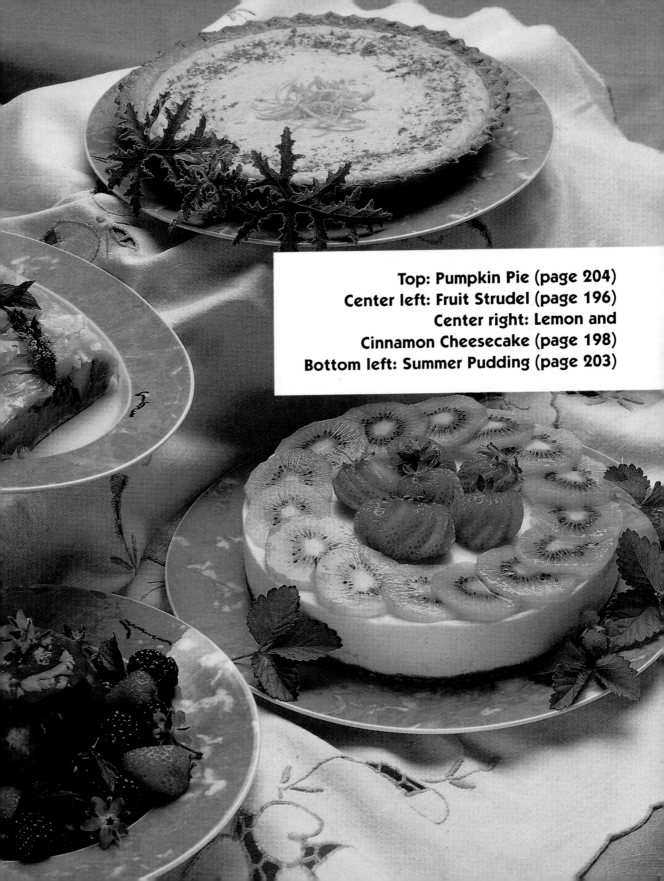

Top: Pumpkin Pie (page 204)
Center left: Fruit Strudel (page 196)
Center right: Lemon and
Cinnamon Cheesecake (page 198)
Bottom left: Summer Pudding (page 203)

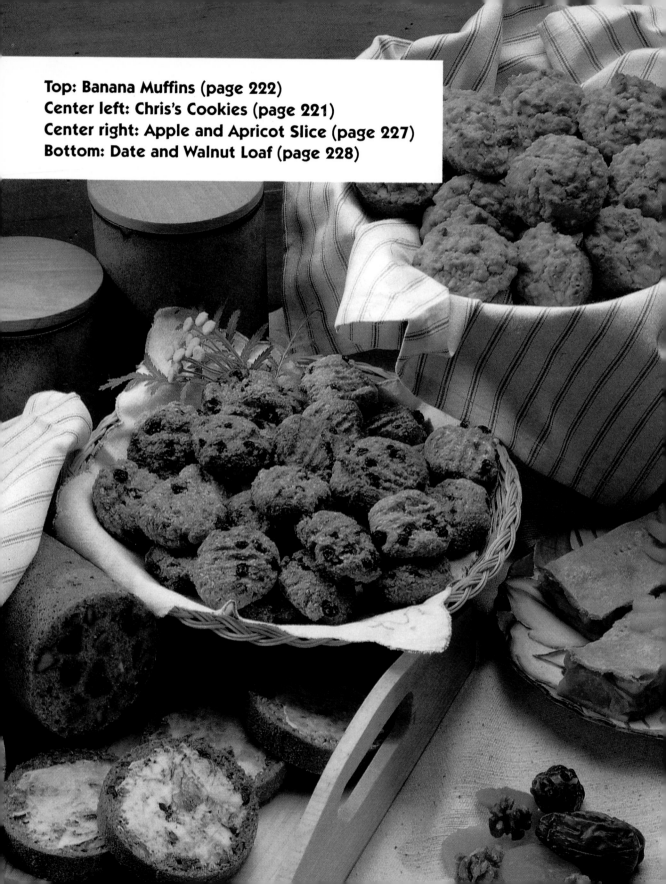

Top: Banana Muffins (page 222)
Center left: Chris's Cookies (page 221)
Center right: Apple and Apricot Slice (page 227)
Bottom: Date and Walnut Loaf (page 228)

Rock Melon Sorbet with Blackcurrant or Raspberry Sauce

Serves: 4

Sorbet:
½ cantaloupe
juice of 1 lemon
1 packet Equal or
 artificial sweetener
 equivalent to 2 tsp
 sugar
Sauce:
1 cup blackcurrants or
 1½ cups raspberries,
 rinsed and hulled
¾ cup water
¼ tsp ground cinnamon
2 tsp cornstarch
1 tbsp water
1–2 packet Equal or
 artificial sweetener
 equivalent to 2–4 tsp
 sugar

The key to a smooth sorbet is in the beating during the freezing process which ensures that the ice crystals which form are small and even.

Sorbet:

1. De-seed and peel cantaloupe.
2. Cut into pieces and blend in food processor or blender until smooth.
3. Add lemon juice and Equal and blend again.
4. Pour into container, cover, and freeze for 2-3 hours until just set.
5. Reblend in food processor or blender or use an electric beater. The mixture should become creamy.
6. Fold in egg white.
7. Refreeze.
8. Before serving, remove sorbet from freezer and allow to soften a little.

Sauce:

9. Place berries, water, and cinnamon in saucepan.
10. Heat gently until fruit has softened and lost its shape. Remove from heat.
11. Make a smooth paste of cornstarch and water and add to fruit, stirring well.
12. Reheat until mixture has thickened.
13. Cool, and add sweetener to taste.
14. Refrigerate until ready to serve.
15. Pour over sorbet and serve.

Nutritional data per serving:
29 Calories, Carbohydrates 7g, Protein 1g, Fat 0g.

Exchanges per serving: ½ Fruit.

Preparation time: 1 hour.
Cooking equipment: food processor, blender or electric beater, saucepan.

Mocha Mousse

Serves: 4

2 egg yolks, separated
13 fl oz full cream
  evaporated milk
1 tbsp cocoa
½ tsp instant coffee
  granules
3 tsp gelatin
3 tbsp water
3 packets Equal or
  artificial sweetener
  equivalent to 6 tsp
  sugar
1 cup light whipped
  topping
Garnish: chopped dates
  or fresh strawberries

This is a scrumptious dessert. Prepare it the day before you want to serve it because it needs to set.

1. Beat egg yolks, and combine them in a saucepan with milk, cocoa, and coffee. Mix until smooth.

2. Stirring constantly, warm the mixture over medium heat, being careful not to boil. Remove from heat and cool.

3. Sprinkle gelatin over water and dissolve over hot water, or microwave on medium for 10 seconds. Cool slightly.

4. Stir into chocolate mixture. Add sweetener.

5. Fold whipped topping into chocolate mixture.

6. Pour into serving dishes. Cover and refrigerate overnight.

7. Serve chilled and garnish with chopped dates or strawberries.

Nutritional data per serving (does not include garnish): 157 Calories, Carbohydrates 14g, Protein 4.5g, Fat 9g.

Exchanges per serving: ½ Whole Milk, ½ Starch.

Preparation time: 45 minutes, plus setting time.
Cooking equipment: saucepan.

Bread and Butter Pudding

Serves: 4

4 eggs
1 pint skim or low-fat milk
2 tsp vanilla extract
3 slices whole wheat bread
2 tsp margarine
2 tbsp raisins
1 tsp ground nutmeg

1. Place eggs in bowl and beat.

2. Add milk and vanilla extract.

3. Spread bread with margarine and cut each slice into four squares.

4. Place three squares in each individual baking dish.

5. Pour an equal amount of the mixture into each dish.

6. Sprinkle raisins and nutmeg evenly into the four dishes.

7. Place the four individual dishes in a larger baking dish, and carefully pour water into the larger baking dish to reach two-thirds up the outside of the individual baking dishes.

8. Bake for 30-45 minutes until set, or arrange the puddings in a wide circle in the microwave to ensure even cooking. Microwave on medium for 8-10 minutes.

Nutritional data per serving:
200 Calories, Carbohydrates 19g, Protein 13g, Fat 8g.

Exchanges per serving: 1 Medium-Fat Meat, ½ Skim Milk, ¾ Starch, ½ Fat, ¼ Fruit.

Preparation time: 1 hour.
Cooking equipment: individual baking dishes, large baking dish for water bath.
Oven temperature: 350°F.

Baked Yogurt Slice

Serves: 8

Crust:
12 whole wheat crackers or 1 cup Meg's Muesli (page 66)
2–3 tbsp unsweetened apple juice

Filling:
1 cup low-fat fruit yogurt
1¼ cups ricotta cheese
juice of 1 lemon
zest of 1 lemon
2 tbsp unsweetened apple juice
2 egg whites
½ cup raisins

1. Grind the crackers or muesli in food processor or blender or crush well with rolling pin.
2. Add apple juice to cracker crumbs to make a spreadable mixture.
3. Line tart tin with aluminium foil and press the biscuit crumb mixture into it.
4. Blend yogurt, ricotta cheese, lemon juice and zest, and apple juice in food processor or blender.
5. Beat egg whites stiffly. Fold them through the blended cheese mixture with the raisins.
6. Pour into cracker base.
7. Bake approximately 30 minutes until firm.
8. Cool and cut into slices.

Variation: Use different flavored yogurt.

To store: Cover with plastic film and refrigerate for up to two days.

Nutritional data per serving:
187 Calories, Carbohydrates 25g, Protein 8g, Fat 6g.

Exchanges per serving: ¾ Medium-Fat Meat, 1 Starch, ¾ Fruit.

Preparation time: 1 hour.
Cooking equipment: food processor, tart tin.
Oven temperature: 350°F.

Christmas Pudding

Serves: 6

4 tbsp white raisins

2 tbsp currants

3 tbsp raisins

zest of 1 orange

1/2 cup grated carrot, apple or cooked pumpkin (or a mixture of two)

3 tbsp brandy

1/2 cup whole wheat flour

1 tsp ground cinnamon

1 tsp mixed spice

1/2 tsp nutmeg

2 tbsp margarine

1 1/2 slices whole wheat bread, crumbed

1 egg, lightly beaten

1/3 cup skim or low-fat milk

1 tsp vanilla extract

2 tsp caramel coloring

1 tbsp brown sugar or Equal

1/2 tsp baking soda

1 tbsp hot water

This is better if made a week before you want to serve it, so that the flavors have time to mature.

1. Soak dried fruit, orange zest, and carrot, apple, or pumpkin in brandy overnight.

2. Mix flour and spices.

3. Rub margarine into flour mixture, and add bread crumbs.

4. Add egg, milk, fruit mixture, vanilla, caramel coloring, and sugar or sweetener.

5. Combine baking soda and hot water and mix well with other ingredients.

6. Pour into a greased bowl, cover securely and steam for 1 1/2-2 hours.

7. Turn out and serve with Custard Sauce (page 193).

To store: Cover and refrigerate. Reheat by steaming or boiling for 30-45 minutes until heated through, or microwave, covered, on high for 5-7 minutes. Do not store it again after you have reheated it.

Nutritional data per serving:
298 Calories, Carbohydrates 46g, Protein 10g, Fat 6g.

Exchanges per serving: 1 1/2 Fruit, 1 1/2 Starch, 1 Fat.

Preparation time: 2 1/2 hours, plus overnight.
Cooking equipment: pudding basin, steamer or large saucepan.

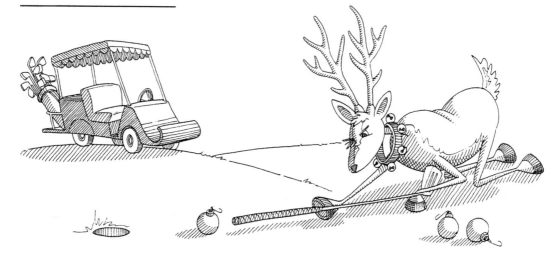

Crunchy Peach Ice Cream

Serves: 6-8

14 oz can solid pack
  pie peaches
juice of $\frac{1}{2}$ lemon
$\frac{1}{2}$ tsp ground cinnamon
1 oz ricotta cheese
3 oz low-fat yogurt
Equal or 2 tbsp apple
  concentrate to taste
2 tsp liqueur (optional)
2 tbsp dried shredded
  coconut
2 tbsp chopped
  blanched almonds,
  toasted
3 tbsp crunchy cereal
  (muesli, puffed rice, etc)

The more carefully you beat the mixture part way through the freezing process, the smoother and creamier your ice cream will be. Homemade ice cream is better used fresh, as ice cream tends to go hard if refrozen.

1. Blend fruit in food processor or blender until smooth and creamy.

2. Add cinnamon, ricotta cheese, yogurt, and apple concentrate; blend well. Add liqueur if desired.

3. Spoon into container. Cover and freeze for 2-3 hours until almost set.

4. Remove and thaw slightly. Break up the ice crystals by returning to food processor or blender, blend until creamy, then spoon back into bowl and add coconut, nuts, and cereal.

5. Fold into ice cream, cover and refreeze until firm.

6. Remove and allow to thaw a little before serving as this ice cream is much more delicious if a little soft.

Nutritional data per serving:
83 Calories, Carbohydrates 7g, Protein 4g, Fat 4g.

Exchanges per serving: $\frac{1}{2}$ Medium-Fat Meat, $\frac{1}{2}$ Fruit.

Preparation time: 1 hour over 1-2 days
Cooking equipment: food processor or blender, mixing bowl with lid suitable for freezing.

Baked Goodies

Whole Wheat Pastry

Serves: 3

1 cup whole wheat flour
1 cup unbleached flour
4 oz margarine
juice of ½ lemon
½–¾ cup of ice water

You can use 2 cups of whole wheat flour if you like, but the pastry will be heavier than the version we suggest here. A food processor is a great help; it turns pastry-making into a quick and easy process, but be careful not to over-process the pastry or it will become heavy.

1. Combine the flours in a large bowl.
2. Rub the margarine into the flour until the mixture resembles bread crumbs.
3. Combine juice and water and add it to the dry ingredients, a little at a time, working it in after each addition, until you have a soft dough.
4. Turn dough onto a lightly floured board and knead lightly. Cover and allow to rest before using.
5. Use dough as required.

Note: Most pastries need to be baked in a hot oven—400°F—for 15 minutes, or until lightly browned.

To store: Wrap in plastic film and refrigerate for up to two days.

Nutritional data per serving:
234 Calories, Carbohydrates 24g, Protein 4.56g, Fat 13g.

Exchanges per serving: 1½ Starch, 2⅓ Fat.

Preparation time: 15 minutes.
Oven temperature: 400°F.

Herby Corn Muffins

Makes: 12

1 cup unbleached flour
1 cup cornmeal
½ tsp salt
2 tsp baking powder
1 tbsp margarine, melted
1 cup low-fat milk
1 egg, beaten
¼ tsp black pepper
½ tsp dried mixed herbs
2 tbsp grated low-fat
  Cheddar cheese

These savory muffins are a great accompaniment to pumpkin or corn chowder. Eat them fresh because they won't keep.

1. Sift flours, salt, and baking powder into a bowl.
2. Mix margarine, milk, and egg and add to dry ingredients. Beat until smooth.
3. Fold in seasonings and cheese, and spoon mixture into lightly greased muffin tins.
4. Bake for 15-20 minutes until golden brown. Turn out to cool.

Nutritional data per muffin:
112 Calories, Carbohydrates 17g, Protein 4g, Fat 3g.

Exchanges per serving: 1 Starch, ½ Fat.

Preparation time: 30 minutes.
Cooking equipment: muffin tins.
Oven temperature: 425°F.

Whole Wheat Damper

Serves: 6

2 cups whole wheat
  pastry flour
3 tsp baking powder
½ tsp salt
2 tsp margarine
⅓ cup skim or low-fat
  milk
⅔ cup water
1 tbsp sesame seeds

1. Sift flour into mixing bowl. Return bran to sifted flour. Add baking powder and salt.
2. Rub margarine into flour until mixture resembles fine breadcrumbs.
3. Combine milk and water, and pour into dry ingredients. Mix quickly, blending with a knife.
4. Turn onto a floured board. Work into a round shape.
5. Place on lightly greased baking tray. Sprinkle with sesame seeds. Bake for 20-30 minutes until brown. Serve warm.

Nutritional data per serving:
183 Calories, Carbohydrates 31g, Protein 7g, Fat 3g.

Exchanges per serving: 2 Starch, ½ Fat.

Preparation time: 50 minutes.
Cooking equipment: baking tray.
Oven temperature: 440°F.

Carrot Cake

Serves: 20 slices

2 cups whole wheat
  pastry flour
3 tsp baking powder
1 tsp salt
½ tsp baking soda
2 tsp ground cinnamon
1 tsp ground nutmeg
¼ tsp ginger
¼ tsp ground cloves
2 cups grated carrot
½ cup shredded coconut
½ cup chopped walnuts
½ cup raisins
2 eggs
¼ cup apple concentrate
1 cup skim or low-fat
  milk

1. Grease and lightly flour cake tin.
2. Sift flour, baking powder, salt, soda, and spices. Return bran to flour mixture.
3. Add carrot, coconut, nuts, and raisins.
4. Beat eggs until fluffy and add apple concentrate. Beat again and add milk.
5. Fold into dry ingredients. Stir until well mixed and pour batter into prepared cake tin.
6. Bake until cooked through (approximately 40-45 minutes).
7. Cool on cake rack.

Variation: Replace walnuts with pecans.

To store: Keep in an airtight container for up to four days.

Nutritional data per slice:
113 Calories, Carbohydrates 16g, Protein 4g, Fat 4g.

Exchanges per serving: ½ Starch, 1 Fat, ½ Fruit.

Preparation time: 1 hour.
Cooking equipment: 8 inch cake tin.
Oven temperature: 400°F.

Pikelets

Makes: 12-16

¾ cup self-rising flour
¾ cup whole wheat
  pastry flour
1 tsp baking powder
¼ tsp salt
1 egg
¾ cup skim or low-fat
  milk
oil for frying

We have given special recipes for conserves and spreads in this book; they are perfect served with these pikelets.

1. Blend flour, baking powder, and salt in basin and make a well in the center.
2. In a small bowl, beat egg and mix in milk.
3. Pour the egg and milk mixture into the center of the flour and gradually beat in the flour using a wooden spoon.
4. Beat mixture well.
5. Heat frying pan and lightly oil.
6. Drop spoonfuls of mixture into pan allowing room for each pikelet to spread.
7. When mixture begins to bubble, turn over with a knife.

8. Let pikelets cook until light brown on each side and lift onto a clean cloth. Keep covered with cloth to keep them soft.

9. Serve with Fresh Strawberry Conserve (page 68), Dried Apricot Conserve (page 66) or Date and Fig Spread (page 67).

Nutritional data per pikelet (if 12 made):
81 Calories, Carbohydrates 13g, Protein 3g, Fat 2g.

Exchanges per serving: 1 Starch, ¼ Fat.

Preparation time: 30 minutes.
Cooking equipment: large frying pan.

Chris's Cookies

Makes: 24 cookies

1 cup rolled oats
1 cup whole wheat pastry flour
1½ tsp baking powder
½ tsp salt (optional)
½ cup rice bran or oat bran
½ cup granulated sweetener
½ cup shredded coconut
½ cup currants
2 large very ripe bananas, mashed
2 eggs, beaten

You can use raisins or chopped dried apricots instead of currants to make these quick and easy cookies.

1. Mix dry ingredients, add banana and eggs, and mix well.

2. Break off small pieces and roll into balls. Place on lightly greased oven trays, and flatten each ball with the back of a fork.

3. Bake for about 15 minutes or until just beginning to brown.

4. Remove from oven trays, and cool on cake rack.

Note: You'll want to make sure your bananas are *very* ripe, otherwise the cookies won't have the right consistency.

Nutritional data per cookie:
117 Calories, Carbohydrates 18g, Protein 4g, Fat 3g.

Exchanges per serving: 1 Starch, ½ Fat.

Preparation time: 25 minutes.
Cooking equipment: 2 oven trays.
Oven temperature: 350°F.

Banana Muffins

Makes: 12

2 very ripe bananas
1 egg
½ cup skim or low-fat milk
½ cup unsweetened apple juice
1 cup whole wheat pastry flour
1 cup white self-rising flour
½ tsp ground cinnamon
2 tsp baking powder
½ tsp salt (optional)

Muffins for breakfast, muffins for school lunch, muffins as a snack . . . muffins full of carbohydrate and fiber.

1. Mash bananas very well. There should be no lumps.
2. Beat egg and add to banana.
3. Add milk and apple juice.
4. Sift flours, cinnamon, baking powder, and salt.
5. Fold flours into liquid mixture. Mix well by hand.
6. Spoon into very lightly greased muffin tins, filling each up by about two thirds.
7. Bake for about 20 minutes until lightly browned and cooked through. Remove from oven, lift muffins out of tins and cool on a cake rack.

Nutritional data per muffin:
112 Calories, Carbohydrates 21g, Protein 4g, Fat 1g.

Exchanges per serving: 1 Starch, ½ Fruit.

Preparation time: 40 minutes.
Cooking equipment: muffin tin.
Oven temperature: 425°F.

Quick Whole Wheat Bread

Makes: 2 loaves, 18 slices each

4 cups whole wheat flour
2 tsp baking soda
17 fl oz plain yogurt
1 tbsp honey (optional)
Topping: 1 tbsp sesame seeds (optional)

This quick and easy loaf contains no yeast, so there is no kneading and rising time required. You can vary the recipe by adding half a cup of roughly chopped pecan nuts or walnuts. Alternatively, try adding half a cup of sunflower seeds or raisins. You may prefer the flavor of the loaf with the addition of a little salt at Step 3, but try it without first.

1. Lightly grease the loaf tin.
2. Measure the flour, unsifted, into a large bowl.
3. Add all remaining ingredients, except the sesame seeds. Use a wooden spoon to mix lightly, but well, until mixture is fluffy.
4. Spoon mixture into the greased loaf tin. Sprinkle with sesame seeds.

5. Bake for 50-60 minutes, or until loaf sounds hollow when tapped.

To store: Keep in an airtight container for up to two days.

Nutritional data per slice:
67 Calories, Carbohydrates 11g, Protein 3g, Fat 1g.

Exchanges per serving: ³/₄ Starch.

Preparation time: approximately 1 hour.
Cooking equipment: 2 loaf tins.
Oven temperature: 350°F.

Blueberry Muffins

Makes: 12

1 cup ripe blueberries
4 tsp brown sugar
2 cups whole wheat pastry flour
4 tsp baking powder
1 tsp salt (optional)
1 tsp ground cinnamon
1 egg
½ cup low-fat berry yogurt
1 cup skim or low-fat milk

They look a little strange, perhaps, but they taste terrific. Eat them fresh; they won't keep. Remember, a trace of sugar will not harm you, particularly when combined with plenty of complex carbohydrate and fiber.

1. Lightly grease muffin tins or spray with cooking spray.
2. Wash blueberries and combine with sugar in saucepan.
3. Heat gently until juice just starts to run.
4. Sift flour, baking powder and cinnamon into bowl. Return bran to flour mixture.
5. Mix egg, yogurt, and milk in a bowl. Add to flour and blend until smooth.
6. Gently fold blueberries into mixture.
7. Spoon mixture into muffin tins, and bake for 15-20 minutes until firm and very lightly browned.

Nutritional data per muffin:
116 Calories, Carbohydrates 21g, Protein 5g, Fat 1g.

Exchanges per serving: 1 Starch, ½ Fruit.

Preparation time: 40 minutes.
Cooking equipment: saucepan, muffin tins.
Oven temperature: 425°F.

Scones

Makes: 12

1 cup whole wheat
  pastry flour
1 cup unbleached
  self-rising flour, less
  1 heaped tbsp
1 heaped tbsp gluten
  flour
2 tsp baking powder
½ tsp salt (optional)
1 tbsp margarine
½ cup low-fat milk
½ cup low-fat plain
  yogurt

The gluten flour used in this recipe is available from health food shops and some supermarkets. The key to perfect scones is to handle the dough quickly and lightly so that it keeps plenty of air in it, and to bake them in a hot oven.

1. In a bowl, combine the flours, baking powder, and salt. Use your fingertips to rub the margarine into the dry ingredients until the mixture resembles fine breadcrumbs.

2. Add the milk and yogurt. Use a knife to work the mixture until you have a fine soft dough.

3. Turn the dough onto a lightly floured board. Using your fingertips, quickly and lightly knead the dough until soft and smooth.

4. Gently flatten the dough to a ¾ inch thickness.

5. Use a scone cutter or sharp knife to shape 12 scones. Avoid rerolling and cutting dough scraps more than once.

6. Place the scones on a lightly greased baking tray. Leave a gap about half the width of a scone between each one.

7. If you want the scones to brown on top, brush each one with a little milk and bake them near the top of the oven.

8. Bake for 8-10 minutes.

Nutritional data per scone:
108 Calories, Carbohydrates 17g, Protein 4g, Fat 2g.

Exchanges per serving: 1 Starch.

Preparation time: 20 minutes.
Cooking equipment: baking tray.
Oven temperature: 440°F.

Variation:

Fruit Scones

Knead 2 tablespoons of raisins, currants, or chopped dates into the dough mixture at Step 2.

Fruit (Christmas) Cake

Makes: 24 slices

1½ cups raisins
½ cup raisins, chopped
2 tbsp brandy
1 tbsp water
1 cup baked, strained
   pumpkin (no lumps)
2 eggs, beaten
½ cup apple concentrate
½ cup skim or low-fat
   milk
½ cup chopped pecans
1 tsp ground cinnamon
1 tsp nutmeg
½ tsp ground cloves
1 cup unbleached self-rising
   flour
1 cup whole wheat
   pastry flour
1½ tsp baking powder
½ tsp salt (optional)
½ tsp baking soda

Apple concentrate gives sweetness to this wonderful fruity cake, and the dried fruit and pumpkin add plenty of fiber.

1. Mix raisins, raisins, brandy, and water, soak overnight.

2. Mix pumpkin, eggs, apple concentrate, and milk.

3. Add soaked fruit, nuts, and spices, then sifted flour, baking powder, salt, and baking soda. Return bran left in sieve to flour mixture. Mix well with a wooden spoon.

4. Spoon into a lightly greased cake tin.

5. Bake 10 minutes at 400°F, then turn down the heat and bake at 350°F until cooked through and browned (approximately 1-1¼ hours). Cool on a cake rack.

To store: Keep in an airtight container for up to 1 week.

Nutritional data per slice:
115 Calories, Carbohydrates 21g, Protein 3g, Fat 2g.

Exchanges per serving: 1 Fruit, ½ Fat, ½ Starch.

Preparation time: 1½ hours, plus overnight soaking.
Cooking equipment: 8 inch round or square cake tin.
Oven temperature: 400°F, then 350°F.

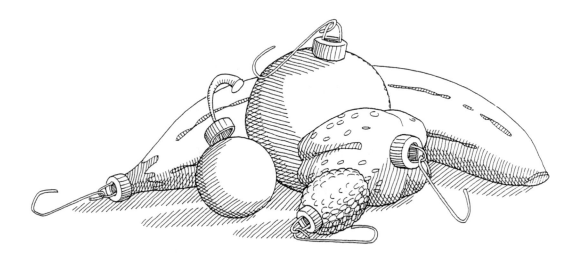

Mince Tarts

You can store any extra filling in a closed jar in the refrigerator for up to two weeks.

Makes: 12

Filling:

½ cup chopped dried
  apricots
1 cup raisins
½ cup chopped pitted
  dates
12 prunes, seeded and
  chopped
6 dried figs, chopped
½ cup slivered almonds
2 apples, peeled, cored
  and thinly sliced
juice of ½ lemon
½ cup brandy
1 tsp cinnamon
1 tsp ground nutmeg
¼ tsp mixed spice
¼ tsp ground cloves

Pastry:

½ cup whole wheat flour
1 cup unbleached flour
4 tbsp margarine
2–3 tbsp ice water
1 egg yolk
few drops liquid
  artificial sweetener

Filling:

1. Combine all ingredients in saucepan.

2. Cook, covered, over low heat until apple is soft. Stir frequently to prevent sticking.

3. Spoon into bowl, cover and refrigerate overnight to blend flavors.

Pastry:

4. Sift flours into bowl, return bran left in sieve to sifted flour.

5. Rub margarine into flour until mixture resembles breadcrumbs.

6. In a cup combine water, egg yolk, and sweetener.

7. Add to flour mixture and stir in with a knife. Turn out onto floured board. Knead lightly, then cover and leave to rest for 10-15 minutes.

8. Roll out dough and cut 12 rounds to fit the bottom of the tart tins. Cut another 12, slightly smaller, to make the lids.

9. Lightly grease the tart tins and line the bases with pastry.

10. Spoon some fruit mince into each.

11. Wet pastry edges and place remaining pastry rounds on top. Pinch edges to seal. Prick tops with fork.

12. Bake for 20-30 minutes until lightly browned.

Nutritional data per tart:
270 Calories, Carbohydrates 43g, Protein 5g, Fat 9g.

Exchanges per serving: 2 Fruit, 2 Fat (mono), ¾ Starch.

Preparation time: 1½ hours, plus overnight soaking.
Cooking equipment: saucepan, tart tins.
Oven temperature: 375°F.

Apple and Apricot Slice

Makes: 16 pieces

1 quantity Whole Wheat
Pastry (page 218)

1 lb fresh apricots, pitted
and quartered or 13 oz
can unsweetened
apricot pieces

3 apples, peeled, cored
and thinly sliced

½ tsp cinnamon

skim milk for glazing

1. Divide pastry into two equal pieces. Roll out first half and cover base of lightly greased cookie tray.

2. Mix fruit and cinnamon and spread evenly on pastry.

3. Roll second half of pastry and place over fruit.

4. Prick surface of pastry with fork or skewer, brush with milk and bake for 30 minutes or until pastry is beginning to brown.

5. Stand on cake rack for 5 minutes, loosen around the edges and flip onto a serving plate. Cool and cut into 16 even pieces.

Nutritional data per serving:
136 Calories, Carbohydrates 17g, Protein 3g, Fat 7g.

Exchanges per serving: ½ Starch, ½ Fruit, 1½ Fat.

Preparation time: 50 minutes.
Cooking equipment: cookie tray, 12 inches x 8 inches.
Oven temperature: 400°F.

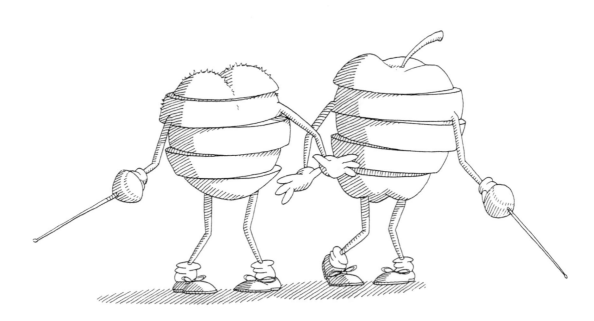

Date and Walnut Loaf

Makes: 10 slices

½ cup boiling water
1 cup chopped dates
1½ cups whole wheat
  pastry flour
2¼ tsp baking powder
¾ tsp salt (optional)
½ tsp ground ginger
2 tsp nutmeg
¼ tsp ground clove
1 tsp ground cinnamon
2 tbsp margarine
1 tbsp sugar
½ cup chopped walnuts
1 egg, beaten
1 cup skim milk

Don't limit yourself to dates and walnuts; substitute any other dried fruit and nuts you choose.

1. Pour boiling water over dates and let stand for 30 minutes.
2. Mix flour, baking powder, salt, and spices in bowl.
3. Rub margarine into flour mixture until it resembles bread crumbs.
4. Add sugar, dates, soaking water, and walnuts to dry mixture and mix lightly.
5. Stir in egg and skim milk.
6. Place in lightly greased nut loaf tin.
7. Bake upright for 45 minutes or until cooked.
8. Leave in tin for 10 minutes before removing to cool.

Nutritional data per slice:
233 Calories, Carbohydrates 35g, Protein 6g, Fat 8g.

Exchanges per serving: 1½ Fruit, ¾ Starch, 1½ Fat.

Preparation time: 1 hour and 10 minutes.
Cooking equipment: nut loaf tin.
Oven temperature: 375°F for 20 minutes, then lower to 350°F for a further 25 minutes.

Whole Wheat Apple-Nut Streusel Cake

Makes: 16 slices

5 oz margarine
¾ cup granulated
  sweetener
3 oz ricotta cheese
1 tsp vanilla extract
3 eggs
½ cup white self-rising
  flour
1½ cup whole wheat
  flour
1 tsp baking soda
1 cup skim milk
1 apple, peeled and grated
¾ cup raisins
1 cup chopped pecans or
  walnuts
½ tsp ground cinnamon

1. Lightly grease and line the base of cake tin.
2. Cream margarine and sweetener, then beat in ricotta and vanilla extract.
3. Add eggs one at a time and beat in.
4. Mix flours and soda and fold into mixture with milk.
5. Add apple and raisins and mix.
6. Spread ½ mixture into cake tin. Add ½ nuts and cinnamon. Spread with remaining cake mixture and sprinkle with remaining nuts and cinnamon.
7. Bake for 1 hour or until cooked.
8. Cool slightly before turning out.

To store: Cover and refrigerate for up to four days.

Nutritional data per slice:
193 Calories, Carbohydrates 15g, Protein 5g, Fat 13g.

Exchanges per serving: ½ Starch, ½ Fruit, 2½ Fat.

Preparation time: 1¼ hours.
Cooking equipment: 8 inch cake tin.
Oven temperature: 350°F.

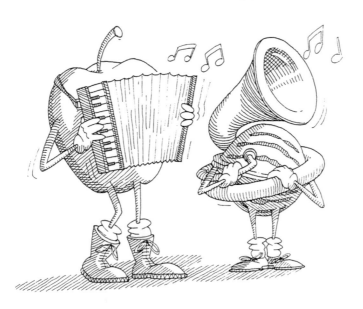

After-Dinner Treats

Fruit Cheese

**Makes: 1 log
approx. 8 inches long**

½ cup dried fruit medley

½ cup hot water

3 tbsp brandy

4 oz each of cottage cheese and cream cheese or 8 oz low-fat cream cheese

3 tbsp poppy seeds

This after-dinner treat can be made one or two days before serving and then be stored in the refrigerator until needed.

1. Place fruit in bowl and add water and brandy. Allow to soak for about 12 hours until fruit is swollen and soft.

2. Drain fruit, retain ¼ cup of the liquid.

3. Blend cheese with the retained liquid until smooth.

4. Stir fruit into mixture and mix well.

5. Tip mixture onto plastic film. Form into a rough log shape approximately 8 inches long. Roll plastic film around log and refrigerate for 1 hour to set.

6. Spread poppy seeds over a clean piece of plastic film and roll cheese log on this to coat with seeds. Return to refrigerator for two hours before serving.

To store: Cover and refrigerate for up to four days.

Nutritional data per serving (4 servings):
252 Calories, Carbohydrates 18g, Protein 11g, Fat 12g.

Exchanges per serving: 4 Low-Fat Meat, 1 Fruit.

Preparation time: 10 minutes, plus 12 hours soaking time and 3 hours setting time.

Rum Balls

Makes: 24

20 shredded whole wheat
  crackers
8 tsp cocoa
5 oz ricotta cheese
3 tbsp unsweetened
  apple juice
2 tbsp brown rum
½ tsp vanilla extract
  (optional)
1 cup shredded coconut

1. Process crackers in food processor or blender until they resemble fine crumbs.
2. Add cocoa, ricotta cheese, apple juice, rum, and vanilla and blend well.
3. Spoon into a mixing bowl, cover and refrigerate overnight.
4. Roll small spoonfuls of mixture in coconut, place on tray and refrigerate.

Variation: Add ¼ cup chopped raisins at Step 2.

To store: Keep in airtight container for up to a week.

Nutritional data per ball:
78 Calories, Carbohydrates 8g, Protein 2g, Fat 4g.

Exchanges per serving: ½ Starch, 1 Fat.

Preparation time: 30 minutes, spread over two days, plus overnight.
Equipment: food processor or blender.

Date Rolls

Makes: 20 pieces

2 cups seeded dates
juice of 1 lemon
½ tsp ground cinnamon
½ cup roasted
  hazelnuts, crushed
4 tbsp poppy seeds
4 shredded whole wheat
  crackers, crushed

1. Blend dates with lemon juice and cinnamon to a thick paste.
2. Add nuts and poppy seeds, and mix well.
3. Form into four rolls, each approximately 4 inches long and 1 inch thick. Roll in crushed whole wheat crackers.
4. Refrigerate for 2 hours, and then cut each roll into five equal pieces approximately ¾ inch thick.

Nutritional data per piece:
75 Calories, Carbohydrates 13g, Protein 2g, Fat 2g.

Exchanges per serving: ⅓ Fat, 1 Fruit.

Preparation time: 30 minutes.
Equipment: food processor or blender.

Frozen Fruit

Serves: 4

8 strawberries, tops left on
20 purple grapes,
    preferably small
½ slice fresh ripe
    pineapple
2 kiwis
Garnish: mint, ivy, or
strawberry leaves

We have used fresh strawberries, grapes, pineapple, and kiwi in this recipe, but you can use any selection of fresh fruit in season. You can also use frozen fruit to garnish drinks.

1. Wash and dry strawberries and grapes.
2. Cut pineapple into eight chunks.
3. Peel kiwi and cut into four pieces.
4. Place fruit on shallow dish and freeze for approximately two hours until firm.
5. Transfer frozen fruit to glass serving plate, and allow to thaw for 10-15 minutes. Decorate with leaves.

To store: Seal in freezer wrap and freeze, if fruit is to be kept more than 24 hours.

Nutritional data per serving:
30 Calories, Carbohydrates 7g, Protein 1g, Fat 0g.

Exchanges per serving: ½ Fruit.

Preparation time: 2½ hours.
Equipment: tray or shallow dish.

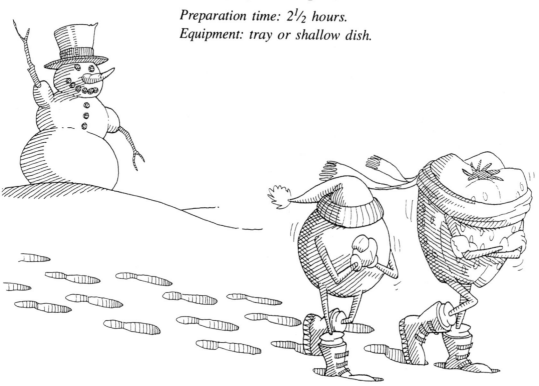

Drinks

50/50 Swirl

Serves: 4

2 cups unsweetened
  orange juice
10 fl oz low-calorie lemon
  drink
lemon peel
orange peel

For special occasions, use chilled champagne instead of lemon drink.

Pour orange juice into a shallow tray and freeze until almost set. Crush and spoon into 4 chilled glasses. Pour half of the lemon drink into each glass and add a swirl of lemon and orange peel.

Nutritional data per serving:
42 Calories, Carbohydrates 9g, Protein 1g, Fat 0g.

Exchanges per serving: $2/3$ **Fruit.**

Orange Buttermilk

Serves: 4

1½ cups buttermilk
1½ cups unsweetened
  orange juice
Equal or other artificial
  sweetener, to taste

Place buttermilk in a jug, then slowly add unsweetened orange juice, stirring constantly. Sweeten with Equal or other artificial sweetener if desired, and pour into glasses over ice cubes.

Nutritional data per serving:
63 Calories, Carbohydrates 11g, Protein 4g, Fat 0g.

Exchanges per serving: $1/3$ **Low-Fat Milk,** $1/3$ **Fruit.**

Strawberry Granita

Serves: 2

Pint of strawberries
1 orange
Equal or other artificial
   sweetener, to taste

Wash and hull strawberries and add to food processor or blender with 8-10 ice cubes and the juice of an orange. Blend until ice is crushed. Add Equal or other artificial sweetener, to taste, then quickly blend again. Pour into glasses.

Nutritional data per serving:
39 Calories, Carbohydrates 7g, Protein 2g, Fat 0g.

Exchanges per serving: ¹/₂ Fruit.

Irish Coffee

Serves: 4

¹/₂ cup whisky
prepared coffee
1 tbsp Creamy Whipped
   Topping (page 192)
Equal or other artificial
   sweetener, to taste

Bring whisky to a boil and simmer for 30 seconds (or microwave on high for 1 minute). Pour into each of four cups, top with hot black coffee and a tablespoon of Creamy Whipped Topping (page 165). Sweeten to taste with Equal or other artificial sweetener.

Nutritional data per serving:
126 Calories, Carbohydrates 2g, Protein 1g, Fat 0g.

Exchanges per serving: 2 Fat.

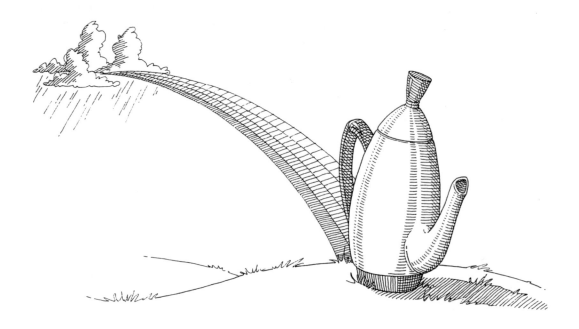

Apricot Cooler

1 14-oz solid pack
 unsweetened apricot
 pieces
½ cup unsweetened
 apricot nectar or
 orange juice
seltzer
mint

Place apricot pieces and unsweetened apricot nectar or orange juice in a food processor or blender. Blend until smooth. Chill well, then pour into four glasses. Fill to top with seltzer. Garnish with mint.

Nutritional data per serving:
44 Calories, Carbohydrates 11g, Protein 1g, Fat 0g.

Exchanges per serving: ¾ Fruit.

Sangria

2 cups claret
½ cup water
1 orange
1 lemon
½ cup unsweetened
 orange juice
Equal or other artificial
 sweetener, to taste
orange slice

Bring claret and water to a boil in a saucepan and simmer for 30 seconds. Thinly slice orange and lemon and place in a jug. Pour claret over the lemon and orange slices and marinate in the refrigerator for 4 hours. Strain the mixture, add unsweetened orange juice, sweeten to taste with Equal or other artificial sweetener, and serve over ice garnished with an orange slice.

Nutritional data per serving:
96 Calories, Carbohydrates 4g, Protein 0g, Fat 0g.

Exchanges per serving: 2 Fat, ¼ Fruit.

Hot Claret Punch

Serves: 4

2½ cups claret
3 tbsps brandy
Equal or other artificial
  sweetener, to taste
nutmeg

Combine claret and brandy in a saucepan or microwave dish. Bring to boil and simmer for 30 seconds, or microwave on high for 4 minutes. Sweeten, to taste, with Equal or other artificial sweetener, pour into glasses and sprinkle with nutmeg.

Nutritional data per serving:
130 Calories, Carbohydrates 2.5g, Protein 0.3g, Fat 0g.

Exchanges per serving: 2½ Fat.

Cherry Shake

Serves: 2

½ cup pitted fresh cherries
¾ cup low-fat milk
¾ cup low-fat natural
  yogurt
¼ tsp ground cinnamon
1 packet Equal or other
  artificial sweetener
  equivalent to 2 tsps sugar

Place cherries in a food processor or blender and blend until smooth. Add low-fat milk, low-fat natural yogurt, ground cinnamon, a packet of Equal or other artificial sweetener, and ice cubes. Blend again until thoroughly combined. Pour into glasses and serve.

Nutritional data per serving:
132 Calories, Carbohydrates 17g, Protein 10g, Fat 3g.

Exchanges per serving: ½ Fruit, ¾ Low-Fat Milk.

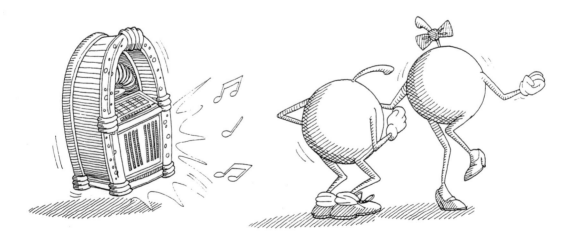

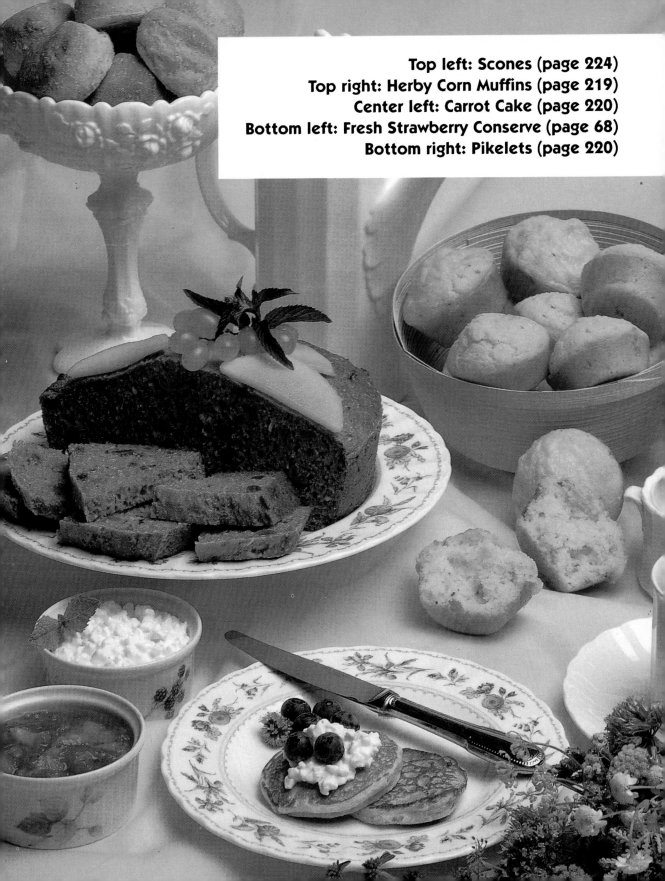

Top left: Scones (page 224)
Top right: Herby Corn Muffins (page 219)
Center left: Carrot Cake (page 220)
Bottom left: Fresh Strawberry Conserve (page 68)
Bottom right: Pikelets (page 220)

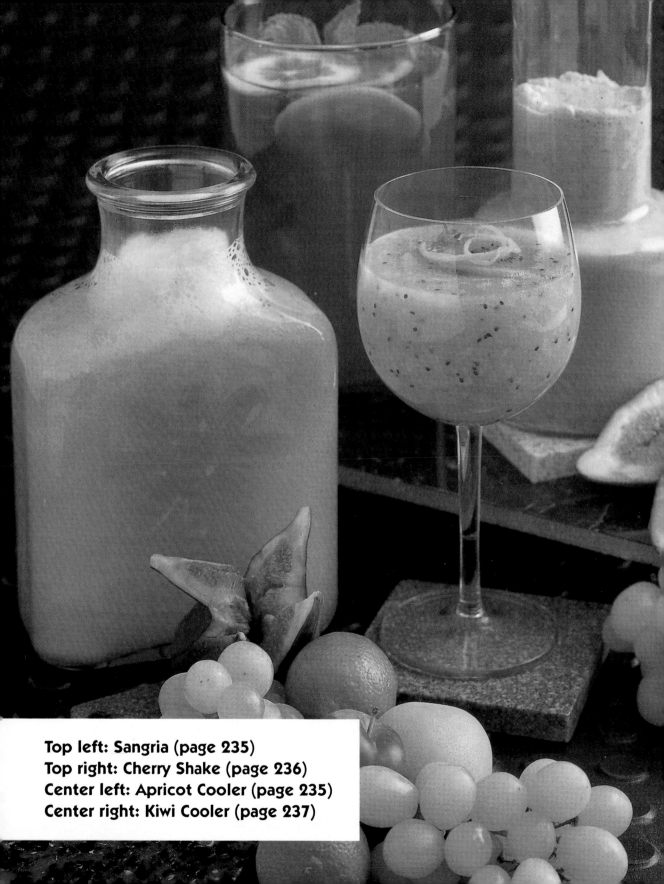

Top left: Sangria (page 235)
Top right: Cherry Shake (page 236)
Center left: Apricot Cooler (page 235)
Center right: Kiwi Cooler (page 237)

Kiwi Cooler

Serves: 4

4 kiwi
2 peeled and pitted
   peaches
2 peeled and chopped
   bananas
2 cups unsweetened
   pineapple juice
sprig of mint

Peel kiwi and place in food processor or blender with peaches, bananas, pineapple juice, and ice-cubes. Blend until ice is crushed. Pour into glasses and garnish with a sprig of mint.

Nutritional data per serving:
129 Calories, Carbohydrates 30g, Protein 2g, Fat 0g.

Exchanges per serving: 2 Fruit.

About the Authors

Christine Roberts is Director of Melbourne Dietetic Centre and consultant to hospitals, commercial organizations, and has a private practice. She has been involved with diet and diabetes for many years, and has co-authored a number of papers. She was a member of the Working Party for Nutritional Resources, Diabetes Australia, in 1988.

She co-authored the successful *Food for Sport Cookbook* and the *Healthy Heart Cookbook* (for the National Heart Foundation). She was also a contributor to Professor Pincus Taft's book, *Diabetes Mellitus*.

Jennifer McDonald is Chief Dietitian at Fairfield Hospital and consultant to a number of other organizations. She has been involved in writing many publications for people with diabetes.

She has co-authored a number of scientific papers dealing with diet and diabetes, in association with other top researchers in the field. Her most recent, *"Temporal Study of Metabolic Change When Non-Insulin Diabetes Changed From Low to High Carbohydrate-Fibre Diet,"* was published in the *American Journal of Clinical Nutrition*, 1988.

Margaret Cox has been involved in both research and clinical work with people with diabetes for many years. For three years she was nutrition coordinator at the Lions International Diabetes Institute, one of Australia's leading diabetes research and educational organizations, and was involved in the development of diabetes education programs and educational resources for people with diabetes.

She co-authored the *Healthy Heart Cookbook* for the National Heart Foundation.

Index